To Trinity Lutheran Church
Library . . . from Trinity
W-ELCA.

Dick Cowen

Papa Raker's Dream

A Loving History of Good Shepherd

by

Dick Cowen

i

This book is joyously dedicated to
Rev. Dr. Conrad W. Raker

ACKNOWLEDGMENTS

My wife Connie quietly and efficiently led me through all my emotional storms in the writing of this book when I repeatedly panicked over simple troubles with the computer. Her skill and knowledge of this electronic wizardry and, above all, her calm were invaluable.

Further, her comments and suggestions in reading the text led to changes that greatly improved the final version.

The encouragement of Anne Gerras of Coopersburg, my literary agent, and her husband Charlie, a senior book editor at Rodale Press, helped so much as chapter after chapter were written. They kept saying, "I like the tone of the book."

Years before this book was envisioned, Randy Kulp, a neighbor of Good Shepherd, read microfilm of old Allentown newspapers for an index of local stories in behalf of the Lehigh County Historical Society. He listed every article on Good Shepherd from 1908 on. That list was a priceless source of material.

Help came also from people at the libraries of Muhlenberg College, Philadelphia Lutheran Seminary and *The Morning Call*.

Lee Berkley at Good Shepherd has been a warm-spirited soul in going over the text on its way to the printer. And it should be also noted that it was development director Lona Farr who initially asked, "Do you want to write a book on the history of Good Shepherd?"

Dick Cowen

TABLE OF CONTENTS

My father was born in a log cabin like President Lincoln. This thought perhaps subliminally had a greater impact on him than many of us realize. And like Lincoln he knew the path upward led through education.

The dream that was to become the dominant force of his life he learned unconsciously at a very early age at his mother's knee. Susan (Dornsife) Raker was a practical pietist who instilled in him the basic Christian virtues of love and compassion. His founding of The Good Shepherd Home can be traced to her deeply etched teachings and personal example. Hard working, but filled with a faith that never wavered, she instilled in him a lifelong devotion to his Lord and His teachings.

Dick Cowen, the author, has admirably traced Papa's life and the early years of Good Shepherd.

As hard as my father worked to make Good Shepherd a reality, it would never have come into being without the industry and attention to detail of my mother, D. Estella Raker. A quiet leader, she was of the same mold as Eleanor Roosevelt.

Possessing a sensitive nature not observed by many, my father said to me, "A man can put up with anything if he has a good home and an understanding wife to come home to." His home was his refuge.

Social legislation of the early Roosevelt years had a serious impact on Good Shepherd, for up to this time we were an orphanage with some handicapped individuals. "Aid to mothers with dependent children" would keep a normal healthy child in the best place for him, at home with his mother. I saw this change coming and began to convert our emphasis to care of the physically disabled.

My father died May 8, 1941. Soon thereafter, I was elected his successor. Within months, World War II was upon us, and all we at Good Shepherd could do was hang on.

Hanging on was more than a phrase. Soon after I succeeded my father, after every mailing of our appeals, hundreds of our blue envelopes would be returned stamped "addressee deceased" or "addressee unknown." These were removed from the mailing list of over 20,000.

It didn't take a genius to know things could go downhill fast. I made appointments to speak every Sunday, and often during the week, always getting new names for the mailing list. Over the years, we built this lifeline up to 84,000.

After the war, we went into a frenzy of activity, expanding in many directions. First the south wing of the Main Building was built. Then there followed the workshop for the handicapped and its expansion. With the help of some Hill-Burton funds from the government, as seed money, the first rehabilitation hospital in the area was built. Soon after, the north wing of the Main Building was gutted and converted into a rehabilitation hospital. Later came the new workshop, formerly a Western Electric warehouse. This building especially appealed to us because the entrance was at ground level, making it accessible to individuals on wheelchairs and crutches.

The true joy of Good Shepherd was seeing Dino Katsiaras, Carl Odhner, Kenny McHenry, Delores Shook, Harry Filer, Clarence Nissley and hundreds of others triumph over their disabilities and become useful, productive citizens and knowing that all of us helped a little.

The Lord has blessed Good Shepherd with thousands of friends. The future looks bright. Tremendous advances are now being made under the guiding hand of our dedicated and energetic president, Dale Sandstrom. Our prayers are that God will continue to bless Good Shepherd as He has in the past.

Dr. Conrad W. Raker

I've taken my approach for this book on The Good Shepherd Home from a lesson Dr. John Raker, its co-founder, learned in 1900.

He had just received a call to be superintendent of the struggling new Lutheran Orphans' Home at Topton, Pennsylvania. The Topton Home had twenty-four children, a new building and a large debt. The support for charity was not as easy as in later years.

He asked a number of persons how to go about the work of meeting the debt and expenses of that home. He personally canvassed most congregations of the Reading Conference. And the answer he got was that he should prepare one great sermon and preach that all over.

He went so far as selecting the text, Matthew 18:5, "And whoso shall receive one such little child in my name receiveth me."

But among other persons, he asked Dr. William A. Passavant of Pittsburgh, the great inner mission champion. Passavant responded, "Little incidents directly from the home will do more good than any sermon you or I, or anybody else, will preach."

After that, John Raker asked a farmer near Topton who replied, "We have our ministers to preach big sermons. When you come around, we want to hear something about the home."

That settled the big sermon question. That sermon was never preached. But the message he spread about life at the Topton Home brought gifts that removed its entire debt in his first year and raised $5,000 for an Old People's Building before he left.

My book on Good Shepherd is something about life in this Home—little incidents directly from its daily existence that hopefully tell something of its mighty work.

Dick Cowen
May 1988

1: FAITH AND FIFTY CENTS

Some brighter day you will
see the Lord's hand in The
Good Shepherd Home as we
see it now.

Sweet Charity
January-February 1909

The Good Shepherd Home was started in 1908 with
"faith and fifty cents." It's been said so often in the
eighty years since that it comes with the ease of
saying "good morning" or "God bless you."

But what prevails is that it's true . . . the faith of the
Rev. Dr. John Raker and his young wife Estella to
establish a home in Allentown, Pennsylvania, for
crippled* children and orphans regardless of race,
creed or color and for elderly, particularly
impoverished preachers . . . and the fifty cents handed
to Papa Raker two years before by James Fritz of Pen
Argyl as the first contribution to what was then only
an idea.

**Editor's note: The words "cripple" and "crippled" have
come into disfavor in recent years. Advocates for people
with disabilities feel that the words that once meant
"deprived of the use of one or more limbs," now carry
implications of inability. In this account of Good Shepherd,
the words are used in their historical sense. It is the
language of an earlier period, a language spoken at Good
Shepherd with love and respect.*

1

Papa had run into Fritz, a member of his first congregation, on a train near Reading. And Papa poured out to him his plan for a home for the most needy. Fritz asked permission to give the first fifty cents to the cause.

It was years later before Papa found out that when Fritz gave him that fifty cents, he didn't have enough money left to get home. Fritz had to walk the final six miles from Belfast to Pen Argyl late at night.

Fritz looked back on that with a sense of pride. "I wish it had been a hundred miles," he said later.

And Papa never forgot where that first contribution came from.

The Rakers began by taking into their Lutheran parsonage one destitute, crippled, thirteen-year-old girl, Viola Hunt of East Bangor, Pennsylvania, on February 21, 1908.

Welcoming Viola was the first tangible step to a "life plan" that had haunted Papa Raker for years. His Lutheran Church had no institution to care for crippled children and infants who were orphans. Yes, if you were over three years old and in good health, there were homes to take you. But not the crippled, not the infants. Two Lutheran orphanages had turned down Viola Hunt precisely because she was a cripple, having had infantile paralysis in her right leg and right arm.

And much as Papa tried to lay aside the idea of establishing a home for what he called the most needy, it returned again and again—like the ghost in Hamlet.

To the Rakers had been born on September 30, 1907, a daughter they named Viola. "No other blessing could have equaled it, with the exception of a little boy," Papa said. "The eager look of her two sisters when they heard her cry for the first time will never be forgotten."

Viola Raker died on December 4, one of five Raker children lost in infancy. She was permitted only twice to enter Grace Lutheran Church where Papa was mission pastor—once for her baptism and four weeks afterward when she was buried.

With the baby's funeral over, and the interment at

2

nearby Fairview Cemetery, the Rakers returned to the parsonage to find one letter.

Again and again as Papa Raker would tell this story across the rest of his life, he would emphasize that the mailman brought only one letter that day. It was an inquiry from Rev. John Henry Miller of East Bangor, asking if there was any provision in the Lutheran Church for a crippled orphan. His particular concern was Viola Hunt from his congregation.

"The name itself had a strange echo in our souls and touched a still deeper chord of conviction," Papa recalled.

And he knew the answer to Rev. Miller's question.

He told his wife that he either had to stop preaching in behalf of orphan children and admit he didn't believe it or take Viola Hunt into their home. Estella was willing if he was . . . and if he was sure it was God's will.

The first Good Shepherd Home was the parsonage, half of a double house, at 630 St. John Street. Papa, Mama, daughters Ruth and Roberta and now Viola Hunt. But not for long.

Within a month, Papa Raker purchased a sprawling farm homestead on the corner just down St. John Street, with three stories and substantial grounds. And by that summer, thirty-seven children and seven old people had applied for admission.

It was his thought to call the home Grace Home for Crippled Orphans and Old People.

Here, another letter intervened, this one from Rev. Jeremiah H. Ritter of Centre Square, Pennsylvania. It was dated March 31, 1908. It read:

"We greatly rejoice to hear of your moving into the new Home and attendant happy circumstances. God be praised.

"I see your letter is without a name for the institution. Here is a suggestion—The Good Shepherd Home for Orphans and Aged.

"Now that you have a ward of Jesus, a Home and applicants for admission, and name, you may be ready to receive further answers to your prayers and faith, and hence the enclosed $5 check towards establishing

3

and maintenance of 'The Good Shepherd Home.' It represents a sacrifice cheerfully and lovingly made."

That was the second donation received for Good Shepherd.

Rev. Ritter had made the first donation to the Topton Orphans Home—$3.74. It was his donation, coming unexpectedly and at a critical period in that institution's history, that inspired its board of trustees to buy a farm at Topton for $7,000 with only that $3.74 in the treasury.

Good Shepherd Home became Papa Raker's ministry for the rest of his life, and he fought for it, prayed over it and shouted its achievements from the housetops . . . and even beyond.

Once, in 1919, after receiving permission from the Allentown police chief, he had copies of *Sweet Charity*, the Home's magazine, and posters dropped from an airplane over Allentown to publicize the upcoming Anniversary Day that August 14. He said that the Lutheran Church shied away from advertising. He had no such reluctance.

And when radio came along in the early 1920s, Papa used that, too.

Conrad (Connie) Weiser Raker, born in 1912, his only manchild to survive infancy, took over when Papa died in 1941 at age seventy-eight. A graduate of Muhlenberg College like his father . . . an ordained Lutheran minister, a graduate of Mt. Airy Seminary in Philadelphia, again just like his father . . . later, the recipient of an honorary doctor of divinity from Muhlenberg, just like his father.

But Connie began as Papa's assistant enriched with academic training his father never had the opportunity for—a graduate year in the social sciences at the University of Pennsylvania with experience that year in jails, hospitals, orphanages and other institutions in the Philadelphia area.

He also brought the familiarity of growing up within Good Shepherd, so much so that as a child he once asked his parents: "How long have I been at the Home?" The cripples and normals of the home were his friends, his playmates, his classmates and,

4

sometimes, his partners in mischief.

Those were the terms then, cripples and normals, and that's what they called each other for decades. The same terms can be heard even now in the conversation of Good Shepherd old-timers. The word *cripples* would eventually give way to terms like *physically handicapped*, *disabled* and the current term, *physically challenged*.

Connie also carried a gentler style than his feisty father.

Papa had fought for survival and won, despite the scoffers and critics in those early years within the Lutheran Ministerium of Pennsylvania, the synod that covered all of eastern Pennsylvania. "O blessed opposition" he would call them in a 1909 *Sweet Charity*. And he would later use *Sweet Charity* to shove some of their own intemperate words down their throats.

He would remind his Lutheran brethren of the struggles the Rev. Uriah P. Heilman had with the Ministerium of Pennsylvania in seeking help to found the Topton Orphans Home a decade before Good Shepherd came into being.

"Synod wished him well, but there was positively no encouragement and enough to discourage almost anyone except Brother Heilman, whose heart was filled to overflowing.

"If synod had to start the Topton Home, there would be no home there today. If starting The Good Shepherd Home had depended on the synod, there would be no Home today," he wrote in 1917.

Oh, Connie would have his battles with the church officialdom—especially in the 1960s when synod attempted to establish a Lutheran United Way, calling for Good Shepherd and other social institutions of the church to give up their own fund-raising and contributor lists and let synod handle it for all.

But for Connie, there was no longer a question of whether The Good Shepherd Home would be. It was.

For Connie, once the austerity of World War II was over, the issue was how great Good Shepherd could become in taking the battered odds and ends of humanity and trying with ever better methods to restore many of them to jobs, to homes, to community, to a renewed sense of worth.

Even in those spartan times of the war years, Connie was quietly changing things . . . redesigning the kitchens so the cooks had fewer steps to walk . . . discarding the dormitory setting for the boys by providing each one with the privacy of his own bedroom area . . . getting higher dining tables so the wheelchairs could slide in under and their occupants be closer to their food.

He would push Good Shepherd in giant steps into national prominence in rehabilitation. He called the construction of the Rehabilitation Hospital in 1964 the greatest event in the history of Good Shepherd since the founding of the Home. And what started as a modest sheltered workshop boomed.

This was no longer a place that served just those who lived within its walls. It had become an outpatient haven for hundreds, thousands. And that workshop business was hardly sheltered anymore. It had sprawled out to include several other locations in the community, and its rallying cry was that it had to be competitive in what it did to stay in operation.

Connie "retired" as superintendent at the start of 1980. Being there every day just got to be too much. "I was sixty-eight. I could see that things were changing and changing fast."

Sadly, the issue of *Sweet Charity* that carried the story on his retirement also included one on the death of his first wife, Hannah. They had been married thirty-three years.

Connie kept his office and continued as a consultant. "I go to see people about helping Good Shepherd, and they respond," he says.

His successor as administrator is the Rev. Dale E. Sandstrom, who had been assistant administrator since 1978. Not a Home boy or even local, but then neither was John Raker. Connie personally chose him. Like both Rakers, Sandstrom is a Lutheran minister.

Sandstrom has presided over a complex that has virtually exploded in the 1980s. Including its workshops, Good Shepherd has become one of the largest employers in the Lehigh Valley.

A three-story Raker Center at Sixth and St. John was opened to house a hundred profoundly disabled people where once the original John Raker parsonage stood. The rehabilitation hospital at Fifth and St. John has risen to four stories where the old folks' building was in the early years.

The small car, plus trauma units served by helicopter medivacs at general hospitals, has brought Good Shepherd a land-office business. "They scrape people off the highways now who used to die," says long-time rehabilitation leader Carl Odhner. "Afterward, they send them to us. Quadriplegics are in and out of here in four weeks."

It is this massive organization that Sandstrom directs. Just the internal telephone directory is overwhelming with its listings for amputee clinic, electrodiagnostic evaluation, ergonomic engineering, scoliosis rehabilitation and a host of other services that require an English translation for most of us.

Ten vice presidents were announced in one issue of *Sweet Charity* in 1986. The ten-thousandth patient at the rehabilitation hospital, Bryan Buck, arrived in December 1982. The fifteen-thousandth, David Leggett, would be there by the fall of 1986. The twenty-thousandth is expected by the fall of 1988.

Sandstrom talks of wholistic medicine, treating the whole person. And what comes from staff meetings is that no matter how big Good Shepherd has become, the constant message is about getting the great majority of patients back in their homes and back in their jobs with their feelings of worth restored.

But this is getting ahead of the story. Let's go back to the Founding Father and the Founding Mother.

You know, for much of these eighty years, John Raker was billed as the founder of The Good Shepherd Home. It's still that way on the inside front cover of *Sweet Charity*.

But take a look at the plaque just put up in 1987 on the front of the Raker Center, named for Connie. It lists the founders (plural) as the Rev. and Mrs. John H.

Raker.

Somebody finally decided to give equal recognition to the woman who was running the place in those pioneer years when Papa was visiting farmers for days in northern Lehigh County to solicit donations of potatoes or was out preaching at Lutheran churches, trying to raise funds and sell subscriptions to *Sweet Charity*.

As a colleague told Papa near the end of his life, "God conferred a very great honor upon you, brother Raker, when he entrusted to you so faithful, so capable and so truly loyal a helpmeet in Mrs. Raker and to you jointly to have Him prompt you and grant you the enabling grace to launch out into the deep." ❖

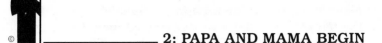

We want to do a few little things well before we die.

Sweet Charity
November-December 1908

John H. Raker was born in a log cabin in a village called Raker in the Mahanoy Valley of north-central Pennsylvania on January 1, 1863, the day Lincoln signed the Emancipation Proclamation. He called it "a most splendid place to be born, but probably not such a good place to remain."

And as he would often say, virtually everything he did in his life until 1908 was in preparation for the establishment of The Good Shepherd Home.

It's the kind of thing people look back on who have a sense of mission.

He would become a scholar of Lutheran Church inner mission history, an adoring fan of Luther, a Christian deeply committed to his work, a bit of a huckster, a yarn spinner and, above all, a champion for the children and old people who came to The Good Shepherd Home. And he would be honored and loved.

He was the fourth child in a family of eleven—six boys and five girls.

His father was a farmer and a gunsmith. He was a great reader, well posted on the topics of the day, but especially on the history and doctrines of his Lutheran Church. He was a stern man and met life stoically, but in the privacy of his home he would get on his hands and knees and play horse with the children.

His pious, God-fearing mother would gather the

children at twilight to teach them their catechism, evening prayers, hymns and Scripture passages.

One evening, she showed the children a picture of Peter and John going up into the temple to pray. At the temple gate, there was a crippled man, begging, who could not walk. Peter said to him: "Silver and gold have I none, but such as I have give I thee: In the name of Jesus Christ of Nazareth, rise up and walk." The man arose and went into the temple, leaping and praising God.

As a child, John Raker said to himself: "Would to God that I might be able to do something like that." And from that day on, his thoughts and efforts would be in sympathy with what he considered the most helpless.

When it thundered, his mother would tell the children that God was speaking. "We were not to be noisy, but to sit down quietly, fold our hands and say our prayers until the storm was over," he would write near the end of his life. "Today, every thunderstorm brings mother's sacred influence and guiding hand back to me to help and to bless."

Professor William Wackernagel, who had John Raker as a student at Muhlenberg College, would recall, "From his youth, he wanted to be a 'good Samaritan,' anxious and ready to render help to his fellowmen in dire need and distress. He was drawn particularly to orphans and homeless old people.

"He is living for the future and is endowed with a good measure of native common sense and practical wisdom."

John Raker during his college years helped Dr. Wackernagel establish St. Stephen's Lutheran Church on what was then the western limit of Allentown.

Once in the early years of the Home, he had to bed down for a time in the YMCA because of a slight case of scarletina within his own household. He admitted how dearly he missed his family, even for such a brief time. "We remember even as a boy, we did not fully appreciate the good qualities of a pocketknife until we lost it."

He also was what we might call today a bit straitlaced.

He was dead set against swearing for anyone, though he forgave it for those who had to drive mules.

That stance probably made him ominously effective when he thundered in a 1917 issue of *Sweet Charity*:

"People do not all have faith in The Good Shepherd Home, nor do all people have faith in our Lord and Saviour. A prominent minister called The Good Shepherd Home a 'bastard' because it was not started as he thought it should have been by the synod or conference. We once heard an unbeliever call the Saviour the same name."

It was the only time that term ever appeared in *Sweet Charity*.

He was totally against drink and tobacco.

As a child, he was in the garden with his mother one day when a young man about sixteen passed the Raker homestead, so drunk he could hardly walk. His mother placed her hand on her son's head and said, "John, I would sooner see you brought home dead than see you come home like that."

He vowed to himself, "Mother, you shall never see that." And he went through life never having tasted strong drink. He wouldn't say it made him better than others, but he was never sorry for it.

During the spring 1889 vacation of his senior year at Muhlenberg College, he was a state speaker in behalf of a constitutional amendment that would make Pennsylvania dry. His college and seminary classmates would particularly recall his vehemence against drink and the seriousness with which he campaigned for prohibition.

The amendment lost five to three statewide. Even in his home county of Northumberland it lost, though only by about 600 votes out of 11,000 cast.

The early readers of *Sweet Charity* would quickly be apprised of his opposition to tobacco. He quoted Luther Burbank on the topic as saying: "No boy living would commence the use of cigarettes if he knew what a useless, soulless, worthless thing they would make of him."

John Raker was a short man physically, five foot

four according to his passport, nearly a head shorter than the woman he married.

He entered the preparatory department of Muhlenberg in 1884 and was graduated from the college in the Class of 1889. Not an honor student, but one determined human being.

He went on to Mt. Airy Seminary in Philadelphia, officially called Philadelphia Lutheran Seminary, Class of 1892. Thus, at twenty-nine, he was a Lutheran preacher.

"We are not entering upon a new work about which we have had no experience," he wrote in the first issue of *Sweet Charity* in 1908. "While attending college and seminary, we already commenced to visit the orphan homes, the alms houses, the hospitals, the prisons, the houses of refuge, the poor, the sick, the friendless, the homeless, the helpless and forlorn, not knowing why we did it. Now, we think we see it plainly. The Lord was preparing us for Our Great Life Plan."

Even as a young man, he was much a renegade. He would become more so as he got older. He often said The Good Shepherd Home followed no beaten path, and the same was true of him.

In the spring of his senior year at seminary, he and his classmate and roommate, Harvey G. Snable, joined surging thousands at the graveside services for Walt Whitman in Camden. They had gone early to make sure to hear Robert Ingersoll, the great agnostic.

He was aware that about a year before the poet's death Ingersoll intended to give a lecture in the Academy of Music in Philadelphia for the benefit of the impoverished Whitman. John Wanamaker, then postmaster general, opposed it because of Ingersoll's attitude against Christianity. The lecture had to be shifted to a hall on South Broad Street.

"We were not delegated by the seminary to attend, nor were we forbidden," John Raker would recall of the funeral. "For some reason, we felt just a little guilty and out of place.

"A friend met us and said, 'I did not expect to see you folks here.'

"We said, 'We did not expect to see you here.' He was superintendent of one of our Sunday schools."

John Raker was a master with words, sometimes with the poetic touch of a Carl Sandburg. Just listen to his concluding observations on that trip to Whitman's funeral:

"Walt Whitman lived in the poorest section of Camden. He loved little children and permitted them to make mud pies on his front doorsteps. When a farmer presented him with a basket of cherries, he beckoned the children to come and help him eat them. A man with such a disposition cannot help but make lasting friends.

"Such was the plain, simple, independent life of Walt Whitman."

John Raker would serve three Lutheran parishes a total of thirteen years and be superintendent for seven years of what is now The Lutheran Home at Topton, Pennsylvania, before he embarked fulltime on the work of The Good Shepherd Home.

His first parish was at Pen Argyl in the slate belt region of eastern Pennsylvania. He would serve seven years, and these years would be recalled for the rest of his life as a most happy time. The people treated him with kindness.

"The blind, the crippled and sickly people were brought to me to take to the hospitals. Just why this was done I do not know. Beautiful, beneficial and lasting contacts were made by doing this," he wrote of his Pen Argyl years.

He went to Holy Trinity Lutheran in Lebanon in the spring of 1898, and it was in that community that he met D. Estella Weiser, tall, bright, stunning, an elocution teacher, sixteen years his junior.

It was the custom of the three Pennsylvania Ministerium churches in Lebanon—Salem, St. James and Trinity—to hold their annual Sunday school picnic together at Pen Ryn, a few miles south of town. In 1898, that day fell on August 25.

While standing with John Reinhold, a prominent layman of Salem, John Raker saw three young ladies run up to a well for a drink. The one in the center especially attracted him and he thought to himself, "There goes my wife if I can get her."

Immediately second thoughts came: "Stop! For all you know that may be a married woman."

Reinhold detected John Raker's interest and introduced Estella, a teacher in the Salem Sunday School.

And John Raker afterward recorded that event in the back of his pastor's pocket-size daybook—the date, the place and who made that introduction. Next in that daybook was a notation that one Estella Weiser was among visitors who attended Sunday services at Trinity that September 1, another that they were engaged that Christmas and finally that they were married June 5, 1899, her birthday.

"The reason we were married so soon was because it was Mrs. Raker's first chance, and I felt it might be my last. So we decided to take no chances and were married on Mrs. Raker's birthday. We would have been married sooner if her birthday had been earlier."

The ceremony was in Trinity. She was twenty, he was thirty-six.

In reporting the occasion, the Lebanon paper would say:

"The bride is one of Lebanon's accomplished ladies, a graduate of Palatinate College, Myerstown, and also of Neff College of Oratory, Philadelphia, and has a large circle of friends. On different occasions, she appeared as an elocutionist in public entertainments and her efforts have been received with much favor."

Palatinate was one of several institutions that subsequently blended into Albright College at Reading.

Neff College of Oratory was established by William Conwell in the late 1880s, just about the time he founded Temple University and created his famous "Acres of Diamonds" speech. John Raker also attended Neff, apparently while at seminary.

The wedding story also noted that the bride was a descendant of Conrad Weiser, the great Indian interpreter.

The bridesmaid was one Hattie Coover, a friend from Lebanon. And among the ushers—all students from Mt. Airy Seminary—was one Ira W. Klick.

14

A decade later, Hattie Coover would marry that Ira Klick, and she would call upon her friend Estella to be in her wedding party. Hattie and Estella became friends for life.

And in 1908, when John Raker was having his troubles trying to scrape up four other people willing to serve with him as the first board of directors of The Good Shepherd Home, one he turned to was the young pastor of St. Stephen's Lutheran Church in Allentown, the Rev. Ira Klick. Pastor Klick said yes.

It seems almost a footnote to the Weiser-Raker wedding to mention that the Rev. Theodore Schmauk, pastor of Estella's church, married them.

Schmauk would later be president of the Ministerium—at a time when John Raker was just a few years into the operation of Good Shepherd. They would have a sharp exchange of views in this later encounter when Schmauk suggested John Raker begin looking for a successor as superintendent. John Raker was indignant. The very idea! He was just getting started.

The Rakers left Trinity in 1900 to run the fledgling Topton Orphans Home, he as superintendent and she as matron. That made them "Papa" and "Mama" Raker as of their arrival that October 1, and they would remain so for the rest of their lives to a multitude of children.

They welcomed Ruth, their first-born daughter, at Topton on Christmas Eve 1900. She would survive at a time many children in the area were being taken to their graves with whooping cough, diphtheria and scarlet fever. The funeral home at Topton that year had just over one hundred funerals, forty-six of them children under five.

Next came a son, Martin Luther Raker, on April 4, 1903. He lived only seven months, and Papa was devastated by his death. How could God do this to him when here he was caring for orphans, the most helpless in His kingdom? Surely, the Lord would spare him the pain of burying his own child.

The day before the burial, Papa, Mama—five months pregnant with her next—and daughter Ruth went together to the newly made grave in the orphans home

15

cemetery to consecrate the ground. In burying Martin, they were leaving a part of themselves there. Four orphan boys were the pallbearers for the funeral.

A daughter, Roberta, arrived on March 10, 1904. She, too, survived and as a young woman would teach at The Good Shepherd Home and direct plays for Anniversary Day. She would marry—in 1931—on the same day her parents did.

It was a shattering experience at Topton, with someone else's child, that would edge Papa ever closer to starting The Good Shepherd Home. It was a story he would tell so many times in the presence of his son Connie that Connie years later could proclaim it from memory—inflections, head-shaking and all.

"While at the Topton Home, we found out something that we never knew before," Papa preached. "We never knew that if a child had lost its father and lost its mother, and in addition to that great misfortune it was crippled or blind or epileptic or sickly, or under three years of age, all our orphanages at that time were closed to such a child."

He cited one such instance to illustrate:

There was a family in Topton by the name of Deaner, the same name as the party from whom the Topton Home farm was bought. This man moved to Chicago. While there, he met with an accident in which he and two sons were killed and the third son lost his right leg above the knee. Another child was born a few months afterward.

The widow now realized she was alone in a great city with a crippled boy and a babe, and the breadwinner had been taken away. She thought of Topton and finally decided to return.

She was disappointed because she found that her brothers and sisters had families of their own, and there was no room here for the crippled boy. She came to Papa Raker with the babe in her arms and the crippled boy at her side and asked him to admit the boy.

"Mother, we cannot receive your boy," Papa said.
"Why not?"
"Because he is crippled," Papa replied.

16

"That is the one reason you should take him."

Then Papa quoted from the charter where it said that "only healthy children between the ages of three and ten, who have all their limbs and senses, can be admitted into this home."

The mother said, "You do not have one child in your home that is as needy as my child."

"Mother, I know it, but I cannot help it."

Papa recalled that something entered his heart and soul from that incident that never left him. And he asked himself: "Has the great Lutheran Church, the church of orphan homes, the church of Francke, Mueller, Bodelschwing and Passavant, the great Church of the Reformation, no home for a crippled orphan child in America?"

And the answer that came back was: "No home."

Papa said the question of the crippled child now became a matter of conscience, and conscience is a stubborn thing. Sometimes, amid thunderstorms and pattering rain, he thought he actually heard the distant cry of crippled children, calling for help.

His first inclination was to accept these crippled children at Topton, but he soon concluded that wouldn't work.

Papa, Mama—four months pregnant with her next— and their two daughters left the Topton Home in April 1907 to come to Allentown where Papa was to serve Grace Lutheran Mission, just south of the city limits.

Papa came with the express purpose of starting a home for crippled children, and he had a proviso on that written into his call. The call stated he could do inner mission work for crippled children as long as it didn't interfere with the work of the congregation.

There was much accomplished in the mission that first year—two catechetical classes, nearly a hundred members added to the church roll and, like at Topton, the debt paid off.

When thoughts came of the crippled child, Papa would say: Some more convenient day.

Viola Raker and Viola Hunt would shortly change all that. ❖

17

Launch out into the deep
and let down your nets for a
draught.

Luke 5:4

"Love will always find its way," Papa Raker wrote in
the first paragraph of the first issue of *Sweet Charity*
in 1908.

"We think we have now reached the practical
beginning of what we are pleased to call 'Our Great
Life Plan.' This consists of preaching and also
practicing the Gospel of Jesus Christ, especially with
respect to the Lord's dependent poor.

"Allentown, Pennsylvania, is the center
geographically, numerically, financially and spiritually
from which this work can be accomplished."

He would go on shortly to say that The Good
Shepherd Home would put Allentown on the map. It
was no boast. It was conviction hitched to an idea.

Work had gone well for Papa in his first year as
pastor of Grace Lutheran mission in Allentown. The
congregation had about sixty members when he
arrived. He added 106 that first year. A debt of $1,250
was paid off. And in the Raker household at 630 St.
John Street, their daughter Viola had been born. The
Great Life Plan was pushed aside to a more convenient
time.

But Viola died in infancy as had Martin before her
and three other Raker children later. Rev. Ira Klick,

then of St. Stephen's Lutheran in Allentown,
performed the funeral service for Viola. The date was
December 7, 1907.

"She had lived for a purpose," Papa wrote.
"Sometimes, we feel that if we had launched out into
the deep with our Great Life Plan—which we believe
the Lord laid on our hearts—we might still have her
with us."

With the funeral service over, the grieving parents
returned to the parsonage to find a single letter in the
mail—from Rev. John Henry Miller of Grace Lutheran
at East Bangor, asking if there was somewhere in the
Lutheran Church to take a crippled orphan from his
congregation. Her name was Viola Hunt. That her
name was Viola was surely more than a coincidence,
Papa felt. It was an omen.

The Rakers said they'd take her into their home.
Viola arrived on Feb. 21, 1908. To Papa, that, too, was
a further sign to sanctify what they had done. It was
the 100th anniversary of the birth of William Loehe,
one of the patron saints of inner mission work.

Viola was born in Pen Argyl in 1894. Papa
discovered later that he had baptized her when she
was ten. Her family moved to East Bangor where the
father died, leaving the mother struggling with six
children. Kind neighbors assisted. Some of the
children were placed with friends.

But Viola, with paralysis of the right arm and leg,
could not be placed anywhere. The Germantown
Lutheran Home said no. The Topton Home said no.

By taking her in, the Rakers had spared Viola from
the Northampton County Almshouse.

"Viola is slow but honest, trustworthy and faithful,"
Papa said shortly after she arrived.

He never said much more about her as a person, no
matter how many times he recounted The Viola Story.

Quickly, Viola was placed in public school. She
would go as far as tenth grade.

But school was something Papa preached
vehemently—that the cripples had to survive in the
real world, and survival lesson number one meant
going up to the end of St. John Street to Jefferson

19

School, whether by crutches or being pulled in a wagon by one of the normals or hobbling onto the trolley car to go out to Allentown High School.

Viola was given instruction in music, too. This again was something the Rakers were to foster and encourage in the children in their care.

After all, Mama had been a teacher in music, elocution and physical culture for four years in Lebanon before she married Papa.

Viola was to stay five years, going back to her mother in 1913 when the mother remarried. Her departure rated only a single sentence—both in *Sweet Charity* and in the board minutes.

Good Shepherd taught Viola to walk, says her daughter, Stella Clark of East Bangor. Mrs. Clark recalls her mother as a kind woman with a good spirit, married to a truck driver, Joseph Counterman, of North Bangor. She bore him twenty-three children, including six sets of twins. Only eight children survived to adulthood.

Viola would return to visit Good Shepherd from time to time on anniversary days, bringing some of her children with her. Her fondness for the Home stayed with her throughout life, Mrs. Clark recalls.

"She loved it. That's how we got to go there to visit. To me, I think it's a wonderful place," Mrs. Clark says.

Viola's death in 1942 was unheralded. It never made *The Morning Call* in Allentown, *The Bangor Daily News* or even the pages of *Sweet Charity*.

Her touch of fame had been her arrival at 630 St. John Street on Feb. 21, 1908.

Meanwhile, the use of that parsonage for The Good Shepherd Home lasted only a short time. If more orphans were to be taken care of, more room was needed. And then there would be added demands with Papa's dreams of taking in needy old people, too, especially destitute retired Lutheran preachers.

These dreams went back to an incident that had occurred while he was superintendent at Topton.

There was a pious mother in the Lehigh County Almshouse who had two fatherless children in the Topton Home. This woman was not old in years, but her suffering made her look old. Papa would visit her to tell her about her children, read God's word to her and pray with her.

While they were praying one day, they were especially annoyed by hearing people nearby cursing and swearing. Papa thought: What if my own mother and father had to spend their last days among such surroundings?

"On bended knee then and there, we promised the Lord that if he would prosper us in our Great Life Plan, we would also do what we could for these pious, faithful old people who did not have enough of this world's goods to pay the admission fee to enter some Christian home.

"This vow is responsible for the fact we take old people at The Good Shepherd Home." And not only did the Home take them, when there were instances of both husband and wife, the Home kept them together—whereas other institutions would split them up into separate quarters.

Papa found a deal for more room, the first of many deals he would swing to expand the physical facilities of Good Shepherd.

As *The Allentown Morning Call* of Feb. 29, 1908, would say under the heading:

SOUTH ALLENTOWN CLERGYMAN
BEGINS A SPLENDID CHARITY

"Rev. John H. Raker, who achieved distinction as the up-builder and superintendent of The Topton Orphans Home, yesterday purchased from Lesher H. Yeager the Tilghman Kline homestead in South Allentown, where he will establish an orphanage for invalid children.

"Mr. Raker left the Topton Home about a year ago to become pastor of Grace Lutheran Church of South Allentown and St. John's Lutheran Church of Fullerton. Since then, he has become impressed with the necessity of a new charity, such as he proposes to establish.

"Mr. Yeager . . . sold the home furnished at a very reasonable price, making a handsome donation in memory of Mrs. Yeager, who died only last fall.

"Mr. Raker, who already has one invalid child under his care at the parsonage, will move to the Kline home at once and will have the orphanage regularly established by April 1. He will appeal to the general Christian public for support."

The name Tilghman Kline already had associations with Lutherans in that neighborhood. In 1897, Kline had donated the site for the Grace mission, though he was not affiliated with it in any way.

The three-story Kline homestead with an acre of ground was at the northeast corner of Sixth and St. John, where the administration building stands. It had nine rooms and a dormitory on the third story.

The price was $7,500. Papa paid $2,000 cash and got a $5,000 mortgage. The remaining $500 was Yeager's memorial gift.

There was a lot of fixing up to be done. People in the neighborhood of Sixth and St. John and others from Fullerton, a village north of Allentown, assisted in cleaning and renovating the place. Carpenters did all their work as a donation. And over one hundred people promised to remember the Home in their prayers.

Papa had a way with getting people to donate their hearts, their skills and their material goods.

For several years, he even got cut-rate electricity for the home from Lehigh Valley Light & Power Co.—until the Public Utility Commission got wind of it in 1914 and put a stop to it.

The local phone company gave the Home free service for about a dozen years before starting to charge. The managers said they would have been glad to continue it, but that the "higher-ups" had objected.

It perhaps would have brought Papa some quiet amusement to read a 1986 *Sweet Charity* item that Bell of Pennsylvania was now providing special directory and operator assistance for people with physical impairments. Those unable to look up phone numbers in the book and those unable to dial would be assisted by operators at no charge.

Besides Viola, another first arrival in the early days of Good Shepherd had a profound effect. She was Aunt

22

Mary (Schindel) Eisenhard, "of blessed memory," as John Raker would say.

She was welcomed at age eighty on November 5, 1908, as the first aged person admitted to Good Shepherd. She had been known as the deaconess of St. Michael's Lutheran Church in Allentown. She was called an "associate" at Good Shepherd and was promptly put to work.

No one in Lehigh County has more friends than Aunt Mary, Papa wrote in announcing her arrival. "It sometimes seems as if she had been either the public school teacher, Sunday school teacher, Mission Band teacher or music teacher of nearly all the mothers in Allentown."

A preacher's daughter, she organized at Jordan Lutheran Church one of the first Sunday schools in that rural area west of Allentown. She taught public school and received two cents per day from each scholar.

Her crowning work was with St. Michael's Lutheran in Allentown. She was a charter member of the church and a leading spirit in the start of its Sunday school. She took an active part in almost everything except the preaching.

In the hall where the first services were held, she used to trim and fill the lamps with oil. Her friends used to tease her: "Aunt Mary, see that the Lutheran lights will not go out for want of oil."

One descendant claims she was probably the first feminist in the Ministerium of Pennsylvania. She helped organize a Women's Missionary Society within the Allentown Conference in the face of opposition from the leadership of the clergy.

At Good Shepherd, she quickly became a regular writer in *Sweet Charity* under the heading "Notes by Aunt Mary." And her picture with the infant "double orphan" Frank May of Reading ran repeatedly in *Sweet Charity*. They were symbols of the young and the old being cared for by Good Shepherd.

It was a touching sight to see Aunt Mary sitting in the midst of children in The Good Shepherd Home, having a little orphan boy on her lap and talking to

23

him lovingly. The old and the young were all together in those early years.

Aunt Mary brought a schoolmarm's charm to her Notes column. Sometimes, she wrote directly to children or to the mothers to tell their children:

"We have a nice yard with all kinds of fruits and shrubbery . . . many kinds of peas, crabapples, grapes, raspberries and pears, which is very nice and handy for the children of the Home, as also for the little companions who come in the yard to visit them. They are allowed to pick the fruit and satisfy their appetites.

"We also have a 'go-cart,' a little carriage, and take the children out riding. Sometimes their little companions come in with their little express wagons and take each other riding."

She noted the "grand success" of the first Anniversary Day, October 2, 1909, and that a motherless child less than four weeks old was admitted on that day. "Although the child is weak and puny, our Heavenly Father will help us love Luella and take care of her. God's will be done."

In another column, she wrote that Good Shepherd was the best home she ever had and that she was blessed to spend her final days there.

Her former pastor, Lutheran Seminary Professor Paul C. Spieker, visited her at Good Shepherd and saw how happy and contented she was and how the Home was prospering. "The Good Shepherd Home has something the Lutheran Church has never learned. It knows how to advertise," he observed.

Aunt Mary died March 30, 1914.

At her funeral, Papa Raker called her one of God's nobility. "She could touch the best that was in a person, and when you give such a Christ-like touch to anyone, it becomes helpful and raises new ideas, new hopes and new life."

Her death didn't stop her column right away. Papa had gone to Aunt Mary several months before her death when she was in failing health and talking about dying and asked her to write some columns in advance. She did.

Her column outlasted her by six months, and it was

obvious from what she said that she knew her friends would be reading her words after she was gone.

There would be other firsts in those beginning years . . . the first Catholic child in the spring of 1910, Emma Schander of Allentown, the first of five Schander children to be taken by the Home . . . the first blind children, sisters Eva, Verna and Anna Pauley of Kutztown, later that same year . . . the first centenarian, Aunt Polly Nauman at age 105 in 1911 . . . the first Jewish child, Lewis Talansky of Palmerton, in 1918 . . . and the first blacks, crippled three-year-old Isabell Younger and her baby brother Philip of Allentown in 1919.

Papa ran a picture of the infant Philip Younger lying in a basket scale on the front cover of *Sweet Charity*. The cutlines declared the Youngers represented the last unfulfilled link in the promise to take helpless children regardless of money, creed, color or nationality. These children had lost both parents to the flu epidemic.

"Some people do not approve of taking colored children. We could not continue to look our Saviour steadfastly in the face and plead the cause of the fatherless and motherless children at The Good Shepherd Home if we had refused to take these helpless children on account of their complexion."

There would be many other firsts at Good Shepherd.

But Viola Hunt and Aunt Mary Eisenhard were the real firsts in a Home that even now never seems to stop pioneering. ❖

The cause of The Good Shepherd Home advertises itself, but we are ardent advocates of printers' ink.

Sweet Charity
November-December 1915

Right from the start, Papa Raker adopted a powerful implement to spread the message of The Good Shepherd Home—a magazine called *Sweet Charity*, published every two months "in the interest of the Lord's poor."

It began with the September-October 1908 edition.

Papa was editor, and retired Muhlenberg College Professor William Wackernagel was associate editor.

The cover featured a drawing of Christ the shepherd, with an angel on each side and a lamb resting on each leg. One angel held a tablet for "Contents" and the other a tablet for "Scripture."

That cover was used for five years. It was drawn by Eugene Carl, the first boy to be admitted to the Topton Orphans' Home.

The listed subscription price was fifty cents a year—a figure that remained the same for sixty-three years.

"*Sweet Charity* will bring a contagious message of love," Papa said. "It speaks in two languages, one to the head and the other to the heart."

And it worked.

It is still working today. The form is far different, so

is the approach. But it continues to tell the message of The Good Shepherd Home—plus The Good Shepherd Rehabilitation Hospital, plus The Good Shepherd Workshops, plus the vast array of other programs out in the community that trace their origins to Good Shepherd.

Papa was known to walk up to an individual and ask, "Have you seen the latest issue of *Sweet Charity*?

"You haven't! Why, you've missed half your life."

And then he would pull a copy out of his pocket and present it.

"The official organ of The Good Shepherd Home goes where you and I cannot go," Papa wrote near the end of his life. "Thousands of dollars have come to the Home through *Sweet Charity*.

"People at the Home do not think much of it and do not help to distribute it as they should. I myself do not think much of it and personally would not give much for it.

"But when I see what wonderful things *Sweet Charity* has accomplished for the helpless, I take off my hat and bow low to this evangel of the Lord."

Just what the circulation was of that first issue isn't clear. But already by the second issue, Papa was claiming that 25,000 people had read the first one. And it wasn't long before he was saying the early issues had become collector's items.

By early 1909, Papa said there were 500 bona fide subscribers, and he was nudging those who had received the limit of three free issues allowed by the postal service. "Subscribe at once or you may get in trouble with the government," he rambunctiously overstated.

In return, he promised to give a true picture of the Home, which would be elevating, interesting and profitable.

"The success of *Sweet Charity* will, to a great extent, make or mar The Good Shepherd Home," he warned.

What he gave his readers for the next thirty-three years was one heaping measure of Good Shepherd—its struggles, its triumphs, its heartaches, its finances

27

down to contributions as small as twenty-five cents, its love.

He also provided one heaping measure of himself— his dreams for Good Shepherd, his doubts, his follies, his zany ideas that worked, his joustings with the officialdom of synod, his obsession with the care of the crippled and the elderly, his love for his work.

And for good measure, Papa, Renaissance man that he was, used his knowledge of the Lutheran Church and the world around him to make *Sweet Charity* also a magazine of social commentary, church history, poetry, humor, prophecy, praise and criticism.

It's eerie to read his piece on Halley's Comet in the March-April 1910 issue. He noted that Aunt Mary was six when the comet last paid its respects to earth in 1835. It was coming by in May 1910, not to be here again for another seventy-five years. "If you want to see this great comet, you better not wait until 1985," he advised.

It's joyous to see his prophetic words from March-April 1912: "It is only a question of time when The Good Shepherd Home must have its own hospital."

It's haunting to come across this mischievous historical observation in the May-June 1922 issue: "In the last forty years, over 3,000 acres of the English coast have slipped into the sea. By this process you can figure out how soon there will be peace in Ireland."

It's heartening to find his courageous words from March-April 1936: "In this country which prizes fair play, colored baseball players are not permitted in the two major leagues."

It's raucous to have him note in the January-February 1912 issue that the Rev. D.G. Wiegner, who recently sold his property to the Home, threw in the outhouse as a donation.

He cited quotations by John Mitchell, the labor leader to the coal miners; jailed Socialist Eugene Debs; Teddy and Franklin Roosevelt; William Jennings Bryan, his personal hero; Booker T. Washington, and the children and old people of Good Shepherd.

He ran Lincoln's Gettysburg Address, Luther's

sermons, Kipling and Elizabeth Barrett Browning's poetry, Helen Keller's essays as well as the gutsy valedictory speech of Luther Schlenker, a Home boy, to his Class of 1935 at Muhlenberg College and a charming essay on the care of a horse that won first prize for Leonard Lohr, a Home boy, in competition with fourteen other fourth-graders at nearby Jefferson School.

When the Home formed a band about 1919 and toured communities and visited churches throughout eastern Pennsylvania to raise money, it was one of the band members, Clarence Nissley, who wrote the account of their travels for *Sweet Charity*. Papa dubbed him "our Horace Greeley" and ran his picture.

Clarence was among the first of many residents to write for *Sweet Charity* and perhaps the most prolific in those early years. Another notable—this one starting with early days of Connie Raker's era—is Carl Odhner, who could have been called "our Will Rogers" for getting a serious message across while still poking fun at himself and his fellow wheelchair users.

Papa also operated a controlled debating society within the covers of *Sweet Charity*. He picked the subjects, of course. He was a participant and also the one reporting on the exchange. But his accuracy apparently didn't bring any screams of foul from his opponents later, and they were people of ecclesiastical stature who would have been heard if they had been wronged.

And he used those debates to prove telling points for the Home.

Take, for instance, some words passed in 1916 between Papa and Lutheran Ministerium President John A.W. Haas, who was also president of Muhlenberg College at the time.

The Home was very much a going concern by then. And the Ministerium, now anxious to have synod representatives on Good Shepherd's board, had been sending a visiting committee for several years to tour the Home and report back to the annual convention.

The feisty Dr. Haas argued that the Home needed the blessing of synod.

Papa countered that Good Shepherd would be doing even better without it, and he noted the Home had never asked synod for a cent.

Dr. Haas: "If the Ministerium would not send the visiting committee to The Good Shepherd Home, the old and staid congregations that have always stood by the Ministerium would not support the Home anymore."

Papa: "Accompany us on a mental trip.

"Let's go to Easton. From St. John's, the largest Lutheran Church in Easton, we have a woman who has Bright's disease, rheumatism and all the ills that human flesh is heir to. She is at the Home practically free—five to six dollars per month.

"Come with me to South Bethlehem. From St. Peter's, the largest Lutheran Church in Bethlehem, we have a woman absolutely free.

"From St. Michael's Lutheran, Allentown, we have two practically free.

"From the Lutheran Church at Emmaus, we took an aged couple, absolutely free. They had thirty dollars and wanted to give it, but the Home did not accept it. The Christian Church should not pauperize anyone.

"The Home also took an aged couple from Macungie absolutely free.

"Go with us to Trinity Lutheran Church, Reading, where the synod met last June. From this church we have an aged person practically free who was a teacher in Trinity Sunday School for over fifty years.

"From Womelsdorf, we have a crippled woman free (this one, however, belongs to the Reformed Church). From Emmanuel's Lutheran Church, Pottstown, we had an aged mother until she died."

Dr. Haas interrupted: "If The Good Shepherd Home is caring for the old members of these rich congregations, why don't you make them pay?"

Papa: "We have a better plan.

"If we charged an admission fee of two, three or five hundred dollars, the congregations or friends would consider that they had paid their obligations, and there it would end. The admission fee might not pay for one year, and yet the persons might live a dozen years or more.

"As it is, the congregations have a debt of love toward The Good Shepherd Home, which we do not believe would be affected by the withdrawal of the visiting committee."

End of debate.

Right in the first issue, Papa instituted a list of those who contributed money to the Home and by the second issue added another listing of those who gave goods.

"We believe in the power of suggestion, and as the Lord's servant we suggest a few things," the first issue proclaimed. He offered a needs list:

"A conference in the coal regions to supply coal.

"Individuals and societies to furnish beds (twenty dollars will secure one).

"Apples, dried and canned fruits of every description.

"Money will furnish many of our temporal needs."

As he mentioned on another occasion, "One of our outstanding rules is not to refuse money."

And right from the start, too, he said he was accepting a promise of help from the Rev. Alfred O. Ebert of the New Tripoli Charge at the northern end of the county. "They will supply the Home with potatoes. This is practical Christianity," he wrote.

The first issue listed these contributors of money, including one woman twice:

Rev. J. Henry Miller, E. Bangor.....................$	1.00
Rev. Jer. H. Ritter, Centre Square.................	5.00
Robert R. Wagner, Allentown........................	1.00
Mrs. Anna Brunner, Coopersburg	30.00
Mrs. Susan Kemmerle, Coopersburg.............	3.00
Grace Lutheran Church, East Bangor...........	17.55
Miss Alice V. Kern, Coopersburg...................	5.00
Grace Lutheran S.S., East Bangor	5.00
Mrs. Anna Brunner, Coopersburg	5.00
A little for the Home, Fullerton.....................	.25
A little for the Home, Fullerton.....................	.25
A little for the Home, Fullerton.....................	.25
Allen Guards O. of I.A., Allentown................	5.00
Dr. Reuben D. Wenrich, Wernersville	25.00

And the "donations received" list in the second issue included:

New Tripoli—J.W. Toy, 2 bushels of potatoes; Henry S. Weaver, 1 bushel; Alvin Brobst, 2 bushels; Nathan Heintzelman, 1½ bushels; Dr. J.A. Kressley, 1½ bushels; W.H. Hoffman, 2 bushels; the Rev. Alfred O. Ebert, 3 bushels; Samuel J. Hartman, 2 bushels.

Moserville—Allen J. Kistler, 4 bushels; Lewis F. Moser, 1½ bushels; Frank Bennecuff, 2 bushels.

That was the start of what the potato farmers of Lehigh County would do for Good Shepherd until it bought farms and grew its own potatoes.

Also on that first donations list was D.D. Fritch of Macungie with two bags of flour.

Fritch supplied the Home with flour year after year. He provided his knowledge as a master farmer to help Good Shepherd when it bought its own farms. He was so good with his advice that one year the Home grew 400 bushels of potatoes on an acre—an achievement that Papa gloried in the rest of his life.

Papa had a feature called "Pregnant Thoughts," single paragraph items, many of them one-liners. Some examples:

—The Rev. Prof. Jacob Fry, D.D., president of the Ministerium, discovered while traveling in the valley of the Nile that babies all cry in the same language.

—You never know human nature if you haven't been in politics.

—On Sunday, October 18, 1908, we preached to the brethren in the Lehigh County Jail. Ninety members and friends of Grace Church accompanied us, and all assisted in the service.

—Lord, give us only enough enemies to keep our friends warm and keep us vigilant, humble and progressive at The Good Shepherd Home.

—God does not always want His children to swim with their heads underwater.

—Our family at The Good Shepherd Home is to be knit together by prayer, faith, love, devotion, forgiveness and good common sense.

—God's dealing with The Good Shepherd Home has been marvelous.

Papa took copies of *Sweet Charity* with him most everywhere he went. He passed them out to passengers on trains. He tried to have a copy put in every room when he stayed at hotels for church conventions—and was usually successful. He arranged for copies to be distributed at the Chicago Exposition and later at the New York World's Fair.

Every few years, he would rerun the story about the traveling man who came across a copy of *Sweet Charity* out in the Midwest, turned around and drove to Allentown to find out what the place was like, left a generous donation and then went home to Michigan to send donation upon donation over the years.

And he liked to tell how in those early times two people left money in their wills to "The *Sweet Charity* Home."

Papa wrote personal biographies of Anniversary Day speakers and prominent Lutheran clergy and laymen—with charm, with feeling, sometimes with humor.

When Allentown Mayor Charles O. Hunsicker agreed to speak at the first Anniversary Day in October 1909, Papa wrote an advance noting Hunsicker was elected that spring at age thirty, the youngest mayor in the city's history.

"If a man has any special faults, they are apt to be magnified during a heated campaign," Papa wrote. "The two most serious charges brought against Mr. Hunsicker were that he was too young to be the mayor and that he was not married.

"He made a campaign pledge and, unlike many candidates, has faithfully fulfilled it. He promises if they gave him a little time, he would soon be older and also get married.

"He is a half year older now and is married for some time already."

Papa carried the obituaries of colleagues, friends, supporters and residents of the Home—again using his knowledge of the individuals to provide a warmth to their final story.

There had been items from time to time about his early years and about the Raker family reunions. But,

33

near the end of his life, Papa used *Sweet Charity* to share more of his recollections of his early life in central Pennsylvania, his college and seminary years. Above all, however, the message was the Home and its residents.

There came a double transition in *Sweet Charity* with Papa's death in 1941.

There was the jolt of his death, though it was not unexpected, considering his declining health that had left him bedfast in those final months. His voice would no longer be heard in *Sweet Charity*.

For eight years after Papa's death, Connie Raker didn't list himself as the editor, not until the September-October 1949 issue.

But there was also the shortage of materials because of the wartime conditions. *Sweet Charity* was to run at times every four months rather than every two to conserve paper. The new message would get out with less frequency.

Connie Raker brought the workers onto the pages of *Sweet Charity*, the people who ran the laundry, those who drove the buses, the maintenance staff, the cooks. What would Papa, the great prohibitionist, have thought of the pages of *Sweet Charity* including a recipe for mince pie by Home cook Salome Strauss that included a stiff shot of whiskey.

Connie had his own skill with words, lines like: "These children every now and then manage to look at the stars."

And *Sweet Charity* under Connie gave the impression at times that the residents had taken over the publication. He had a coterie of talented writers living in the Home who went delightfully wild on its pages—Morris Blinderman, Jack Daubenspeck, Delores Shook (now of "blessed memory") and the irrepressible Carl Odhner and the charming Betty Ruth Pumphrey, plus the artistry of Eric Andrews, another of "blessed memory."

Odhner, for instance, went off with his wheelchair to H. Leh & Co., a department store in downtown Allentown, to interview store executive John Henry Leh for a *Sweet Charity* story on why he had paid for all the shoe-repair work for Good Shepherd residents for years.

The newly formed Good Shepherd Alumni Association had a column of its own in Connie's years.

He broke tradition on something that went back to Papa's first issue—a listing of those who gave money or goods. It had gotten to the point in the late 1940s that in a twelve-page issue, eight pages were devoted to a list of contributers, set in agate type. That took up more space that could be used to tell more of the story of the Home. And that small type skyrocketed the cost of publication.

With board approval, Connie cut out the listings, something perhaps that only Papa's son could have done so swiftly. Virtually no one complained, and the cost of publishing *Sweet Charity* was trimmed by two-thirds, far more than Connie estimated.

Sweet Charity concentrated its view on the Home itself. It no longer was a magazine, in part, of Lutheran Church history, of local church and clergy doings at conference or synod or of Raker family history.

There was also the fact that Connie Raker was and is a private man, whereas Papa was one to spill much of his life out onto the pages of *Sweet Charity*.

When Connie at age thirty-five married Hannah (Ely) Jacks in 1948 in St. Michael's Lutheran Church in Allentown, it was local page news in Allentown's *Morning Call*, something virtually unheard of for a local wedding. That was something ordinarily for the "women's pages."

At the Home, soon after the event, the children were told to gather in the chapel "to meet the governor." Instead, they were introduced to the new Mrs. Raker. As one Home boy remembers it, one of the kids said, "Big deal. Where's the governor?"

And Mama Raker stopped neighbor Randolph Kulp one day just after the wedding: "Well, Randolph, now that Conrad is married, you're the only bachelor on St. John Street. We'll have to do something about that."

But *Sweet Charity* carried nary a line about the marriage.

And it was more than two years later before *Sweet*

Charity first mentioned Hannah. She just quietly began appearing on the pages of the magazine—at an appearance before the alumni association, as an officer in the Ladies Auxiliary, in the crowning of the king and queen at the annual winter ball.

Connie took the stance that he was not the story. The Home was. Rehabilitation was. The idea of a sheltered workshop was. And so were the people who made it work day after day . . . the doctors, the nurses, the therapists, the counselors . . . and the board members and other community leaders who helped raise the money and the industries and service clubs that pitched in.

The text was breezier, more white space between the lines, larger type. Pictures abounded. After all, there was an explosion in magazines and then television to compete for the reader's time. The message had to be given quickly and easily, and it was a rapidly changing message.

The normals were going. As Papa Raker had preached right from the beginning, the effort should be to place them in private homes.

Some of the cripples were being mainstreamed. Papa Raker preached that right from the start, too. That's why he wanted the Home right there on St. John Street, right in town where the cripples could make their way up the street to Jefferson School or struggle on the trolley to get to high school across town.

The live-in quarters for workers were being phased out. And by the time Connie would step down as administrator in 1980, the old people would be gone. After all, the government and just about every major religious body had sponsored housing for the elderly— the poor elderly, those of moderate means and the rich.

And, oh, how Papa Raker lamented the need for places for the elderly.

So the Good Shepherd message was changing. Outpatients were coming in by the dozens and then the hundreds, the thousands. Few if any of the severely handicapped persons who still lived at Good Shepherd were writers who could take to the pages of

Sweet Charity, as could a Carl Odhner or a Clarence Nissley, and become personalities and virtual members of your reading family for a generation.

That is what much of *Sweet Charity* is under Dale Sandstrom's administration, too. The programs of Good Shepherd are the message—what they do for stroke victims and their families, what they do for those getting rehabilitation for broken limbs and their families.

Conrad Raker is still listed as the editor. But the responsibility for the writing rests with full-time staff people who seem to be saturated with a love for the place.

Their task is harder to personalize so that readers still have a warm feeling about Good Shepherd and a firm belief in its mission.

A writer can absolutely wallow in the fun of telling how a young Carl Odhner sang "Without a Song" from his wheelchair at a talent contest in 1948 at Dorney Park, an amusement park just outside Allentown. He took first place among a hundred contestants and brought back to Good Shepherd the grand prize, the first television set the Home ever had. What ecstasy at the Home over this conquering hero!

And that triumph was just a small segment in a joyous saga of Carl's life that would extend across the pages of *Sweet Charity* for decades, even now.

But in this eightieth anniversary year of Good Shepherd, how do you convey the miracles of recovery for those rehabilitated who are in and out in weeks or are outpatients around for just a few hours a week?

It's still with stories of individual patients. But the stories can be no more than brief glimpses into their lives. Those patients are often back home by the time their stories reach *Sweet Charity*'s readers.

The mission of Good Shepherd has moved increasingly to the more severely handicapped. And that has provided a tougher challenge for those who explain that mission to the nearly 100,000 families now receiving *Sweet Charity.* ❖

In the years to come, we will
not be known by what
people did for us, but by
what we did for people.

Sweet Charity
November-December 1912

There was a time in the history of Good Shepherd
when it was not considered much of an honor to be a
member of the board of trustees. The whole idea of
Good Shepherd was regarded as the dream of a short-
lived visionary. This was supported by predictions
from critics that the sheriff would sell the place by the
end of the first year.

Papa Raker maintained that Mama was the only
friend he had who was willing to be a partner in this
venture at the beginning. And his trek through
Allentown and environs throughout most of 1909 to
assemble a board of trustees provides the evidence of
that. He had promised incorporation by that spring.

When the Kline homestead had been purchased in
March 1908 at the northeast corner of Sixth and St.
John streets, Papa was the one to buy it. There was no
corporate structure.

He had been in the lumber business and apparently
done well at it before he studied for the ministry.
While at Topton, he used some of those business skills
to help found the Topton National Bank. He said his
pay as a pastor never matched what he had earned in

lumbering. He had a bit of money, plus good credit, and that enabled him to buy the Kline property.

The law said a charitable corporation had to have at least five members on its board of trustees. Papa felt a small board would be more progressive than a large one. But he had a second reason. He thought he'd have trouble getting even five directors, and he was right.

Robert W. Kurtz, head bookkeeper at Lehigh Valley Trust Co. for many years, and the Rev. Ira W. Klick, then pastor of St. Stephen's Lutheran Church in Allentown, both had shown special interest in inner mission work when Papa was superintendent of the Topton Orphans' Home. Both said yes to serving on the Good Shepherd board.

Gerhard C. Aschbach, who had a music store in downtown Allentown, showed great kindness to the Home by furnishing beds and in many ways helping the cause.

Papa went to see Aschbach in March 1908. Aschbach was at the shore. Weeks passed before Papa got to see him and more weeks until his answer came back: He would do anything within his power for the Home, and he faithfully kept that promise to the end. But he said his business and his health would not allow him to give the time needed to be a trustee.

A friend suggested Professor George T. Ettinger, the dean of Muhlenberg College, to be president of the board. Papa asked him, and Dr. Ettinger asked for time to consider. Then the good doctor sent a beautiful letter saying it would be impossible for him to take up the extra work that the position would entail.

Papa was equally unsuccessful with jeweler Herbert Keller, physicians Willard D. Kline and Eugene Kistler, clothier Harvey Bastian and John N. Lawfer, the proprietor of a carpet store.

Others were considered but not asked because they let it be known they would not accept.

Some skeptics prophesied the Home would never be incorporated, that Papa would just hold onto the property for a certain time and sell at a handsome profit.

39

Fall 1909 came and still no incorporation.

Papa concluded there had been enough delay, that even if it meant taking two other people only temporarily, he had to get the Home incorporated. He prided himself on being a man of his word.

Mama would be the fourth member, so far all Lutherans. But if the Home should desire state aid, Mama could resign and make room for one who was not affiliated with the Lutheran Church.

One more to go.

Papa asked the retired Rev. Dr. William Wackernagel, one of his former professors at Muhlenberg, to be the other temporary member.

"The doctor promised on the condition it would not involve him financially. It seemed all were afraid of the finances," Papa wrote.

Three preachers, Mama and bookkeeper Kurtz. All Allentonians. All Lutherans.

But before the board was organized, a friend advised Papa that it would be better to have more laymen. This friend suggested Leonard Sefing Sr., seventy-one, someone Papa called "the great orphan man of the Lehigh Valley."

Sefing was a noted builder—such Allentown structures as Grand Central Hotel (which became Hess Brothers and later, Hess's, at Ninth and Hamilton), the Lyric Theatre (now Symphony Hall) on North Sixth Street and the Breinig and Bachman Building at Sixth and Hamilton, whose exterior is artistry in brick and whose fourth floor is graced by the tiled heads of buffalo, bulls and other animals.

But, more important, Sefing brought his abilities as a longtime director of the Lutheran Orphans' Home at Germantown and someone much involved in the Lutheran orphanage at Topton. Superintendent Jonas O. Henry at Topton was his son-in-law, married to Sefing's daughter Ida.

Dr. Wackernagel gracefully stepped aside, saying Sefing was just the man because he could settle any misunderstanding among Germantown, Topton and Good Shepherd.

Sefing cheerfully accepted.

The board organized—Papa as president, Sefing as vice president, Rev. Klick as secretary, Kurtz as treasurer and Mama as matron.

Then came a meeting with attorney Marcus C.L. Kline to prepare the necessary incorporation papers for court. Four directors were present. No Sefing. He sent word that he could not serve because of objections from both the Germantown and Topton orphanages.

Dr. Wackernagel to the rescue again. He came at once and, as Papa told it, the first meeting was held on the curbstone at Sixth and Hamilton.

"We rejoiced," Papa wrote. "We had five persons who were willing to identify themselves as members of the board of trustees of The Good Shepherd Home."

And soon after, he posed to his *Sweet Charity* readers this thunderous declaration:

"The question has been asked: Who called this board into existence?

"We unhesitatingly answer: The Lord Himself.

"Just as He called his twelve Apostles, just as He called Nathaniel under the fig tree, just as the Holy Ghost called us through the Gospel and enlightens us by His gifts and sanctifies and preserves us in the true faith, so we believe He called the members of the board of trustees of The Good Shepherd Home of Allentown, Pennsylvania.

"We believe that He still calls and leads men and women as of yore.

"Here we are, constrained, ready, willing and anxious to work in the neglected part of the Lord's vineyard—for the crippled orphans and infant orphans, where the priests and Levites have become accustomed to pass by on the other side.

"We ask you, dear reader, to play the part of Aaron and Hur and hold up the hands of the board of trustees, so that this, the Lord's cause, may prevail, so that we may prove to an unbelieving world that the Lord still hears and answers prayers."

Amen.

Dr. Wackernagel only promised to serve until a suitable replacement could be found. But he quickly became much involved as chaplain of the Home,

41

visiting two or three times a week, preaching an English and German sermon to the old people every Sunday and instructing the children in Sunday school.

He stayed on the board the rest of his life. He died in 1926.

Within a few years, it was easy to get board members. But you need a special kind of individual at Good Shepherd, Papa said, not better than other people, but the right kind for this peculiar work. "We often see zeal without knowledge where churches and institutions are started and afterwards go to nothing," he said.

The board was self-perpetuating like other permanent institutions. Proper selection of the board was vital to the success of Good Shepherd, Papa maintained. And he would shortly report that the board was working harmoniously. "The one great thought has been the welfare of the helpless," he said.

"The Saviour could be present at all the board meetings, and His guidance was and is continually sought. Here is one of the great secrets of The Good Shepherd Home's success."

The charter that went to court said the Home was formed "for the purpose of providing a Christian home for crippled orphans, infant orphans, destitute children, old people and aged or disabled ministers."

It would transact its business at the northeast corner of Sixth and St. John streets in the newly created Twelfth Ward of Allentown.

The five subscribers were also the original members of the board, listed in alphabetical order. "Of these, at least four shall be members of the Evangelical Lutheran Church, three of whom must be members of congregations belonging to the Evangelical Lutheran Ministerium of Pennsylvania and Adjacent States."

The superintendent had to be an ordained Lutheran minister belonging to the Ministerium.

And the provision that showed just how humble were the humble beginnings of Good Shepherd read:

"The yearly income of the corporation, other than that derived from real estate, will not exceed the sum of $20,000."

As the eightieth anniversary nears, the Home spends about $78,000 a day throughout its entire corporate structure, including nearly $17,000 just on the permanent residents.

Judge Frank M. Trexler approved the charter on November 9, 1909.

The trustees also put on the books a constitution at the time, which repeated the name, the intent and the members of the founding board. The terms were staggered from one to five years in this order— Wackernagel, Klick, Kurtz, Mama Raker and Papa Raker.

Officers were to do what officers are expected to do in most organizations. And those provisions carried an assumption made by most organizations—that the ones carrying out those duties would be males.

The great attention in the document, however, was upon the mission of the superintendent, the matron and any teachers—the people who had to run the place from day to day.

SUPERINTENDENT

"The superintendent shall be the pastor of the Home, conduct the devotional exercises, instruct the children in religion and perform all pastoral duties," the segment for Papa began.

There were provisions that the superintendent oversee the employees, inspect the place regularly, keep a journal of worthy events, compile records on each guest and send any money received to the treasurer.

The superintendent was to handle Good Shepherd's correspondence "in his endeavor to keep the Home before the churches.

"He shall see further that the children are trained to habits of industry, order, cleanliness and economy. He shall inspect every article and take care that nothing unsound or improper be admitted into his department . . ."

What's not included is one of the major jobs Papa had—to go out on every highway and byway to solicit money, goods, services and prayers just so the Home could survive.

MATRON

"The matron shall have the immediate care and superintendence of the domestic affairs of the institution and shall at no time be absent from the premises without the permission of the superintendent.

"She shall in connection with the superintendent direct the domestic arrangements, instruct the girls in the various branches of domestic industry, take charge of clothes and bedding and shall particularly endeavor to unfold to those under her charge the advantages of a moral and religious life."

Besides all the seriousness this section carries, it also almost sounds like Mama couldn't leave the place to go buy a pair of shoes without Papa's permission.

TEACHERS

"The teachers in addition to their school duties shall aid in the management of the institution and report offenses and cases of delinquency by the inmates to the superintendent.

"They shall instruct the children in such branches of education as may be required by the school committee, use all proper means to inspire them with a love of study, lead them justly to estimate the value of a sound practical education and constantly strive by precept and example to impress upon them the importance of good order, self-government and purity of body and mind."

They had to make sure the children were prompt. "See that no waste is suffered," teachers were admonished.

* * *

Among other features of the constitution was one that said board members could be removed by their colleagues for "immorality, dishonesty and expulsion from church membership."

Applications were to be made to the superintendent or other board member, after they had been approved by the pastor or church council of the congregation to which the applicant belonged. The board had final say.

Entrance fee for the aged was first listed as $300. But the board could permit exemptions and "each case shall be considered upon its own merits."

That changed in 1914 to simply say that "no fixed entrance fee shall be established and each case shall be considered on its own merits."

That was pretty well the way Papa had been doing it right from the start anyway.

He would repeat in *Sweet Charity* over the years the details of an early board meeting when the trustees were faced with admitting an old person with $7,000 and another soul who had nothing. The Home desperately needed the money. There was room to take only one. And the first inclination of the board was to take the one with the $7,000.

But then Wackernagel asked: "Who is most needy?"

The answer was obvious, and the board voted unanimously to accept the one who had nothing.

The original constitution said if any aged inmate arrived with more than the amount required for admission or came into money afterward, the board was to invest the excess and give the inmate the interest for the rest of that person's life. The principal went to the Home when the person died.

The aged guest was to be on probation for six months. "An aged inmate becoming dissatisfied shall at any time be at liberty to leave the institution." And the board had the power to dismiss any aged guest if the welfare of the Home required it.

The board actually had to resort to dismissal of a guest in several instances in the early decades. One was a troublesome retired Lutheran minister, who was transferred to the state hospital where he died soon after. It was torment for Papa to turn out this fellow member of the cloth and further anguish when the man died.

Finally, the constitution provided for an advisory

board and auxiliaries.

It directed the trustees to appoint the advisory board, originally twenty-five to thirty persons, later increasing the possible maximum to forty, to meet once a year, inspect the property and offer suggestions on ways to improve.

It said the creation of auxiliaries was desired to aid the board to properly furnish and maintain the Home and provide clothing for the inhabitants.

An Allentown Auxiliary was already a fact for nearly a year before the board constitution was created.

The auxiliary was founded August 26, 1909, at a meeting at the Home. Miss Laura V. Keck of St. John's Church was president, Mrs. Robert W. Kurtz of St. Michael's was the secretary and Mrs. R.S. Diehl of Christ Church was the treasurer.

The advisory board, all males, didn't surface on the pages of *Sweet Charity* until the fall of 1912. There were nine laymen and twenty-one clergy.

The laymen were:

Gerhard C. Aschbach, music dealer, Allentown.

August M. Brown, druggist, Auburn.

Paul A. Eben, cashier, Metropolitan Life Insurance, Reading.

Allen P. Leibensperger, contractor, Fullerton.

William M. Mearig, traveling salesman, New Holland.

Edward E. Miller, lawyer, Lebanon.

Edward Raker, lawyer, Shamokin.

Capt. H.M.M. Richards, treasurer of American Iron and Steel Manufacturing Co., Lebanon.

Joseph D. Wagner, post office clerk, Sunbury.

The clergy:

M.J. Bieber, General Council field missionary, Toronto, Canada.

Alfred O. Ebert, pastor of New Tripoli Parish.

Charles L. Fry, pastor of Trinity Church, Catasauqua.

George Gebert, pastor of Zion Church, Tamaqua.

A.J.D. Haupt, Albert Lea, Minn.

Edgar J. Heilman, president of the Danville Conference, Elizabethville.

Edwin F. Keever, president of the Lutheran Synod of

New York and New England, Utica, N.Y.

Prof. Elmer F. Krauss, Lutheran Theological Seminary, Chicago.

George C. Loos, city missionary, Brooklyn, N.Y.

Prof. Frank P. Manhart, Selinsgrove University.

Solomon E. Ochsenford, pastor of St. John's Church, Bath.

Adam L. Ramer, superintendent, Slav Missions of the General Council Lutheran Church in North America, Allentown.

John C. Rauch, pastor of St. Luke's Church, Allentown.

Wilson M. Rehrig, pastor of St. John's Church, Mauch Chunk.

Jeremiah H. Ritter, pastor of Mildred Parish.

Nelson F. Schmidt, pastor of Schwenksville Parish.

H.M. Schofer, pastor of Mahanoy Parish, Red Cross.

H. Douglas Spaeth, pastor of St. Mark's Church, Williamsport.

S.A. Bridge Stopp, supply pastor, Allentown.

Joseph Stump, pastor of Grace Church, Phillipsburg, N.J.

Elias A. Yehl, pastor of Trinity Church, Bangor.

Papa had one simple rule for membership on the advisory board. You had to first visit the Home.

Papa didn't really put the advisory board members to use collectively until the fall of 1914 when he sought their advice and endorsement on the idea of buying farms.

By then, there were already ten ladies' auxiliary units besides Allentown—those in Bethlehem, Birdsboro, Coopersburg, Harrisburg, Hegins, Mauch Chunk (now Jim Thorpe), Quakertown, Reading, Sellersville and South Bethlehem.

Meanwhile, the constitution for the Home's board was adopted May 13, 1910.

The basic legal paperwork was now completed for what already was a going proposition. ❖

There is a little doubt
connected with everything
we do for the first time and a
little sadness with everything
we do for the last time.

Sweet Charity
March-April 1918

When you open a business, you first have to get a
good location. And for Papa, Sixth and St. John streets
in Allentown's South Side was an excellent spot.

"Over 5,000 people pass The Good Shepherd Home
every day," Papa observed in 1908 in the second issue
of *Sweet Charity*.

The Home was right there in the real world, not
hidden off in some corner of the countryside.

And Papa was off and running, living the motto that
"the more you expect, the more you are likely to get."
He pushed ahead for more and better in behalf of the
orphans, the cripples and the aged in his charge. He
showed little fear of debt. His financial credit was
astounding, and he was a master at raising money—a
skill he had already demonstrated at Topton Orphans'
Home and Grace Church in Allentown where he was
still pastor.

The opening issues of *Sweet Charity* also showed
how successful Papa was at recruiting talented people
to help with the cause. They carried a column listing

the professional and commercial people whose services he had already lined up to help . . . three physicians; a dentist, eye doctor and music teacher; two lawyers (one being Papa's brother Edward in Shamokin); a florist, baker, barber, tailor, shoemaker, justice of the peace and freight hauler.

"The superintendent, matron and all others mentioned in this column cheerfully render this work of love at The Good Shepherd Home free of cost for the Lord's poor," *Sweet Charity* explained.

Papa would work as superintendent for several years without a salary. What he did receive was his pay as pastor of Grace Church up the street. At the end of 1909, the board did put Mama on the payroll. Her salary as matron was established at $15 a month.

Papa transferred the Kline homestead at the northeast corner of Sixth and St. John to The Good Shepherd Home corporation in 1909 for what he paid for it, $7,000—plus the taxes. About $1,000 in improvements had been made.

That transfer put the Home in debt for $8,000 within a year after it was founded.

But Papa pointed out that a conservative real estate agent had put the value of the property at $13,000.

Papa appealed to the public through *Sweet Charity* and the public press to wipe out the debt. He was never bashful in asking for your soul and your pocketbook. He came courting in behalf of the orphan infants, the cripples and the elderly, and he told you right out how he was going to sweep you off your feet.

"What we need first and foremost in this great work of the Lord is your heart, your sympathies and your prayers.

"If we secure these, then you will become a living fountain and cheerfully and continually help and give for the orphans' cause and, thus, work not only for time, but also for eternity and experience those sweet stirrings of the soul, and God's eternal sunshine will settle in your heart and home."

And Papa grabbed at your heart with stories like the one about Frank May, the one he called the "double orphan," the first infant taken into the Home.

Frank came from Reading, a baby his parents didn't want to care for. "The child would have starved to death if it had not been for the Associated Charities of Reading that supplied him with milk," Papa said.

Frank was three times in Reading Hospital in his first year. Attempts were made to secure a place for him in a private home, but no one would take him. The agent for a child-placing society turned to Good Shepherd.

The board agreed to take Frank, and he arrived October 1, 1908, wrapped in swaddling clothes. He was eight days short of a year old. He weighed twelve pounds. He could not hold his head up.

Papa said that a prayer formed in his mind comparing this child to the birth of Christ in the manger: "This little child is also wrapped in swaddling clothes. There is no room for it at the inn. No one loves it. No one wants it. Help us to love it and bring it up in the nurture and admonition of the Lord."

When the person who brought the baby left, Papa and Mama went into the room where this helpless little child was lying on the couch. Papa locked the doors. He remarked how repulsive the child was to look at and acknowledged that wasn't the proper spirit for foster parents to have. "We want to see behind this child the dim outlines of our Blessed Saviour and to hear Him again say, 'Suffer the little children to come unto me' . . ."

There was a rap at the door, a minister calling. He walked to the couch and said, "What do we have here?"

Papa replied, "This little child has just been brought to the Home. We have not had time to change and wash its clothes."

The minister stood for a few moments and then said with emotion, "If you will take care of that little child, I will stand by you and help you."

And when the preacher left, Papa repeated the great verses from Matthew and Mark that called for the caring and loving of children and the doing of humble works.

Mama, four months pregnant, picked up the baby,

pressed him to her bosom and commenced to love him as her own.

Frank thrived. His weight nearly doubled by Christmas.

Papa wrote, "And when he left the Home two years later, he had so ingratiated himself in the hearts of all that there wasn't a dry eye in the Home. There was something in this child that was divine."

Papa had a little financial footnote to his story. Frank was there just as long as he needed help. When the child had a family that wanted him, then he left—"to make room for another needy one and make a dollar do double service."

* * *

John Yost of Wescosville and his sister Theresa (Yost) Gilbert of Allentown can share the meaning of Good Shepherd from within the Home in those early years. They lived it as orphaned children.

They were normals.

"We were by far better off at The Good Shepherd Home than if we have been in our own home. We were educated. You learned to stand on your own two feet. We could do everything," Theresa says.

"Mama and Papa Raker were like mother and father to us. They would always give you a second chance.

"You couldn't have had a better home. If anybody should have been Mother of the Year, it should have been Mama Raker."

John was eight and Theresa six when they arrived in 1915.

The parents had had a farm about ten miles southwest of Allentown. Both were dead, the mother of tuberculosis, leaving four children.

Good Shepherd only had room for two, John and Theresa. A brother was admitted to the Topton Orphanage and then was adopted by a Mennonite farm family in Lancaster County who worked him hard. And a twelve-year-old sister went out on her own, working in a hotel north of Allentown.

John and Theresa came to Good Shepherd

sponsored by St. Peter's Lutheran in Allentown, though the minutes don't specify which St. Peter's (there are two).

"I cried for a week," John recalls of his arrival at Good Shepherd. "Aye, aye, aye, they took pity on us. We had an uncle and they got us to live with him. But he had five of his own. So they sent us back to Good Shepherd. Then, we got accustomed."

Mama never hit the children. But Papa often sent John down the cellar to await a paddling when he was bad. "Sometimes he forgot about you and never did come down. And, yes, his son Conrad got paddled like the rest of us."

John says there were rodents to battle in the old Kline homestead. One he captured and kept for a time in a jar. And it was his duty to make the trips to the ground cellar for foodstuffs because others were fearful of what wildlife they would encounter.

Kids from the neighborhood would take meals with them. And when there was mischief in the area, "we Home kids were always blamed for a lot of stuff we didn't do," John says.

Theresa remembers one time being punished at catechetical class up the street at Grace Lutheran, where the Rev. Phares G. Beer was pastor. The kids all referred to him among themselves as "Piggy Beer," a takeoff on his first two initials, P.G., Theresa recalls.

"He made us learn and recite 'A Mighty Fortress' as punishment. It was no punishment at all because we already knew it from all the services at the Home."

John says, "As kids, we didn't have any money. The police would come out at Christmas and you'd get ten brand new pennies. I thought a lot of those pennies.

"And you got ten cents a day for working on The Good Shepherd Home farm. They'd take you out of school for two weeks in the fall to help pick potatoes."

Papa would load them up in his touring car, boys and girls, for the trip out to the farm that has long since been a part of Allentown's park system. He would call out, "All aboard for Schickshinny," which was a place near his childhood home.

Theresa says that when she got to high school and

took German, a retired German preacher at the Home helped her with her translations. "Then, the other kids copied from me," she recalls with a smile.

Clarence Nissley, one of the disabled young men who went on to college, seminary and graduate school and then came back, used to write Theresa's English essays for her. "They knew darn well at high school I didn't write them."

John left in 1925 to join the Navy when they had coalburners, and he shoveled a lot of coal. Primarily, he served as a carpenter, a skill he had developed at Allentown High School. "The Home wanted to send me to Lehigh University," he says. But he made the Navy his career for twenty years, rising to chief carpenter's mate.

He was at Pearl Harbor on December 7, 1941, on the Sacramento, a gunboat. "I saw the Oklahoma turn over, and I saw the Arizona blow up. It was lucky our battleships were in rather than our carriers. If the carriers had been there, the war would have lasted two more years."

After the war, he retired and soon after that married Mary Schander, one of the first Catholic children at the Home. He is a recent widower as the Home's eightieth anniversary approaches.

His sister Theresa finished high school in 1931. The Ladies Auxiliary of the Home paid for everything when she went on to nurses training at Lankenau Hospital in Philadelphia, and Papa put her picture on the cover of one issue of *Sweet Charity* to proclaim her achievements.

She married, worked at a private hospital in Allentown for a number of years and then shared the responsibilities with her husband in a television and radio business for thirty-three years. She is a recent widow.

Sweet Charity carried bits and pieces of their life at the Home and then as they went out into the world. They are among a few from those early years who are still around to tell their doings themselves.

* * *

The story of the three blind Pauley sisters spreads across twenty-five years of Good Shepherd's early history. They arrived at the Home on April 4, 1911, three weeks after their mother died. Their father and the Rev. Robert Lynch, pastor of Trinity Lutheran in Kutztown, brought them.

Eva May, five years, Verna Alverta, three years eight months, and Anna Louisa, ten months. A two-year-old sighted brother went with grandparents at first, then later to the Topton Orphanage.

The Good Shepherd Home board minutes noted, "The poor authorities have pledged $1.25 per child a week until sixteen years old toward their support."

Papa came to the girls' defense immediately on the pages of *Sweet Charity*.

"Many people have said to us that these children should be taken to a home for the blind. There is no home for the blind. We have schools for the blind, but no home.

"The school for the blind will receive them when they are six years of age, but only for the school term. In other words, they must have a home that will supply them with clothes where they can go during vacation.

"The Good Shepherd Home will give them a home and do all for them that medical care can do. After a while, people will see the great necessity for a Home like The Good Shepherd Home."

Anna Louisa was placed in the infants' cottage, among fifteen tots cared for by Sister Mable Stanley, a deaconess from the Baltimore Motherhouse. The baby died of pneumonia within a year.

Papa said her funeral was as sad as the death of "little Nell," but all felt it was better for little "Anna" to be with the Lord than to remain in darkness at The Good Shepherd Home.

The Home would be in operation for almost ten years before Papa could report to the board that it had finally gone through a year without the death or serious illness of a child.

Eva and Verna Pauley were nearly always together. But in the fall of 1912, they were separated. Eva was enrolled in the Overbrook School for the Blind in Philadelphia. Verna became restless: "I call for Eva, but she does not answer me."

When Eva returned for the Christmas holidays, the blind sisters would be seen sitting together, holding each other's hands, talking, singing and as happy as they could be. But Verna's sadness resumed when Eva went back to Overbrook.

As Papa told the *Sweet Charity* audience, many have experienced being homesick sometime in childhood. Imagine what it must be like to have blindness added to that.

He promised Verna that she would be the next admitted to Overbrook, so she could be with Eva again. And he was a man of his word.

Those first ties of Good Shepherd with Overbrook branched out in many directions. When other blind children at the school had no place to go for the holidays or for the summer, the Home took them in—a very present help in trouble.

Papa soon came to hail Eva as "our Helen Keller."

As the sisters grew, they had a part each year in the anniversary program. Sometimes, they sang a duet. Sometimes, they joined to sing with others who were crippled in other ways.

And as they learned Braille and acquired a Braille Bible, Papa saw in their skills yet another way to extol the achievements of the Home. He had them read from the Braille Bible at the 1921 Anniversary Day.

He reported afterward, "When the blind girls read the simple story of God's word from the raised letters on Anniversary Day, the large audience was moved with compassion. They saw and 'remembered them that are in bonds.' They looked into the closed eyes of the readers and listened to the messages and messengers as if they came from another world.

"An awe and silence fell upon the audience which was akin to the Divine. It was a touch of the day of Pentecost."

Verna contracted tuberculosis in the spring of 1922 and died in Allentown Hospital that November. Papa and Mama were with her the night before she died.

"Verna was a beautiful Christian character," Papa said.

Sweet Charity carried a letter Eva wrote of her to Mama and Papa in the fall of 1923 from Overbrook: "It is now nearly a year since Verna is gone to the Promised Land. It seems so different without her.

"We used to play together and tell each other interesting stories that we made up ourselves, and what fun we did have. It seems I talk about her in every letter I write to you, but I cannot help it."

And in 1924 a letter from Overbrook to Mama and Papa, also shared with *Sweet Charity* readers, Eva said:

"I have a little favor I would like to ask of you, Papa Raker. Would you this Easter take me to see my brother? And as you know, I have never been to my sister's grave since she passed away. Would you mind taking me there sometime?"

And in 1925, Eva wrote: "Do you still have the children of our Home broadcast over the radio?

"I remember at Christmas time when I told the Christmas story over the radio, and when Florence (another blind girl) and I sang.

"I like to do things for you, because you have done so much for me and also because I know and can feel that I am doing it for my dear Christ."

Eva's letters, Papa's notes about her and a picture published several times of Eva at a typewriter made this young woman virtually a member of every *Sweet Charity* family.

At the Home's twenty-fifth anniversary program in 1933, before the traditional Braille readings of Matthew 25:31-46 and the thirteenth chapter of First Corinthians, the chapter on love, she offered this prayer:

"Precious Lord, bless the portion of Thy Word which is to be read on this our great anniversary occasion. Bless these thine own dear people who are gathered here for the sole purpose of serving Thee. May the good seed sown fall into good ground, bringing forth fruit a hundred fold in the hearts of all hearers.

"Let a double portion of Thy blessing fall upon the

founders of our Home, and if it be Thy most holy and gracious will, grant that many more new friends may be added who will gladly carry on the wonderful work of serving love toward all mankind."

Tuberculosis struck Eva in her final years and lingered as it had for Verna before her. Her last days were spent at Hamburg State Hospital, a place that specialized in TB treatment. She died in February 1937.

A generation of *Sweet Charity* readers had lost a dear friend. ❖

God bless and prosper this
Home with all its friends and
inmates. Amen.

Aunt Mary's Prayer.

Papa Raker thought big.

He may have been scrounging for survival in those
first years of The Good Shepherd Home—asking
housewives to fill canning jars with foodstuffs,
knocking on the doors of farmers at the northern end
of the county for donations of bushels of potatoes,
urging individuals in the Wilkes-Barre Conference to
help contribute toward a freight car load of anthracite.

But he wasn't long into the operation of The Good
Shepherd Home before he was talking of the time the
Home would spend a million dollars a year.

He had the Rev. Frank N.D. Buchman, just back
from a visit to the Holy Land, as the guest speaker for
the first Christmas Day service in 1908 when the
Home was just a handful of people. Buchman was a
Sunday school pupil of Aunt Mary's, a Muhlenberg
classmate of Papa's brother Frank, the same Buchman
who would later lead the controversial Oxford
Movement and still later the international Moral
Rearmament organization.

Fifty-five attended. The choir of Grace Church sang.

Buchman would return to speak the next three
Christmases and then send $100 from China a few
years later.

Papa secured as guest speaker for Anniversary Day 1911 the director of the Russell Sage Foundation in New York.

Sage had left a multi-million-dollar estate to his widow, and she had established the foundation, its prominent feature being a "child helping department."

Foundation director H.H. Hart told Good Shepherd's 1911 anniversary assemblage: "You are here laying the foundations for an institution that may stand for 500 or 1,000 years and may involve the expenditure of millions of dollars."

At that time, the population of the Home was fifteen infant orphans, eleven crippled orphans (three being blind), three old ladies and one aged minister.

Papa asked President Wilson to come to speak at the Anniversary Day program in 1913. He said the President was especially interested in crippled and blind orphan children. Papa shared his exchange of letters with *Sweet Charity* readers. He wrote:

"Encouraged by your practical Democratic simplicity, we venture to ask you without the influence of a lobby to give a short address at the Fifth Anniversary of The Good Shepherd Home, Allentown, Pa., on Labor Day, Monday, September 1, 1913.

"It would be just like you, after having been elected to the highest office of the nation, and of the world, to stop by the wayside, like the Good Samaritan, in behalf of the most helpless orphan children, the crippled, the blind and the sick infants.

"Enclosed you will find a program of our last year's anniversary, also a few cards showing the nature of our work. Blessed is the nation whose God is the Lord. Psalm 33:12.

"Waiting for a favorable answer, we remain your humble servant."

J.P. Tumulty, Wilson's secretary, replied, saying the President directs him to acknowledge "your kind letter and thank you for the cordial invitation. He regrets, however, that he is unable to accept, for the reason that he is declining all invitations to attend public functions during the first year of his administration."

That brief Tumulty reply was enough for Papa to put

this optimistic heading over the exchange of letters:
"EXPECT PRESIDENT WILSON AT NEXT YEAR'S
ANNIVERSARY OF THE GOOD SHEPHERD HOME."

After all, there was the word "hope" in that phrase
"faith, hope and charity" in the thirteenth chapter of
First Corinthians that Papa loved so dearly. And
Tumulty had only said no for 1913, hadn't he?

Papa tried again in 1914, this time enlisting the aid
of Congressman A. Mitchell Palmer of Stroudsburg,
later to be attorney general in Wilson's second term.
Papa ran a copy in *Sweet Charity* of Palmer's letter to
the President. But, alas, this came to naught.

The President's ailing wife Ellen died on Good
Shepherd's Anniversary Day 1914. Papa sent a letter
of condolence to a loved and honored President:

"The crippled and blind orphan children, as well as
the aged and helpers in The Good Shepherd Home,
join me in extending their heart-felt sympathy to you
and pray the Lord to sustain you and yours in the
hour of your great bereavement.

"Mrs. Wilson was a model wife and mother for our
nation and the world.

"The fact that Mrs. Wilson died on the day of our
anniversary, the day we had hoped to have you with
us, made a deep impression on us all."

The White House responded with a note saying that
"the President and the members of his family
acknowledge with grateful appreciation your kind
expression of sympathy."

Papa resigned as pastor of Grace Church, effective
the last Sunday in April 1911, to become
superintendent full-time at Good Shepherd.

"For four years, we have walked together as people
and pastor in the ways of love and peace," he wrote to
the members of Grace Church. "The dissolution of a
pastoral relation so close and tender seems to me now
the most painful voluntary act of my life.

"You all know that the Lord's work at The Good
Shepherd Home has grown to such an extent that it is
absolutely necessary for the superintendent to devote
more time to the work at the Home. For this reason
and this alone, I now resign as pastor of Grace

Church."

He served the Home without pay as superintendent in those first years and his family was crammed into two rooms in the Kline homestead. With his resignation from Grace, the Home board gave him a salary of $50 a month and his keep.

Papa got the board to acquire more properties, quickly.

Retired Prof. William Wackernagel, the old man of the board, told the first training class for Christian workers for the Home: "I see great prospects, brethren. I see these buildings enlarging and multiplying. I see these gates widening as the years roll on."

That message was delivered October 19, 1910.

And, by then, Papa had already given Wackernagel some concrete evidence.

What was called an infants' cottage had been purchased down the street from the Kline homestead on August 4, 1910. And Papa had a centurion band formed in the Danville Conference to pledge the money for the project and for its improvements over the years.

It was not a cottage, really, but a three-story brick house next door to the homestead. The cost was $4,000—with alterations and improvements.

Papa would record later in *Sweet Charity* that "some would-be social worker" said he didn't understand what Papa was doing by having the crippled, blind, sickly babies and old people altogether in the Kline homestead.

"Like the mother who thought her boy should learn to swim before getting into the water, some thought we had no business to take such persons until we had the proper building to care for them." And he admitted that old people and little children did not suit together, especially without the proper facilities and help.

But he reasoned that if the public saw the great need of separate buildings for the babies and the old people, the Home would be able to secure them. And he had been using the pages of *Sweet Charity* beforehand to enlighten the public to that great need.

61

The next great need was a separate building for the old people and the nurses when not on duty. A new three-story brick building that was erected for a hotel at the corner of Fifth and St. John was purchased for $7,450 in April 1911.

Papa had quite a bit to do with making that property less than attractive as a hotel. He opposed a liquor license for the place. Lehigh County Court Judge Frank Trexler agreed, turning down applicant Rudolph Heske in March 1911 because the establishment "is too near The Good Shepherd Home, the management of which remonstrates."

Then a lot was acquired for $1,200 on St. John Street, leaving only one property in the entire block not in Good Shepherd hands. That was a double house, brick, purchased in May 1914 along with some nearby lots for $16,100.

The total meant property worth over $55,000 with a debt of $22,500.

And then came the farms. ❖

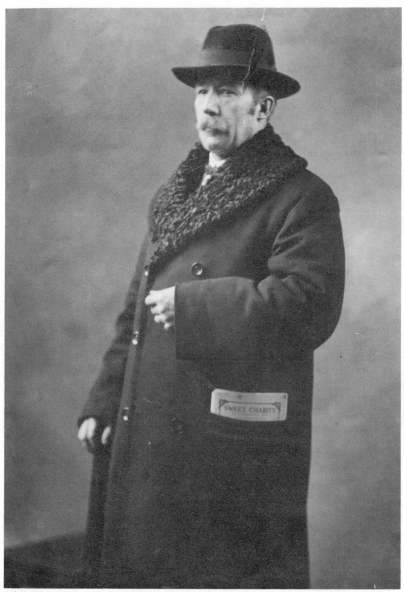

The Rev. John H. Raker, superintendent of The Good Shepherd Home, 1908-1941, with Sweet Charity *magazines in his pocket.*

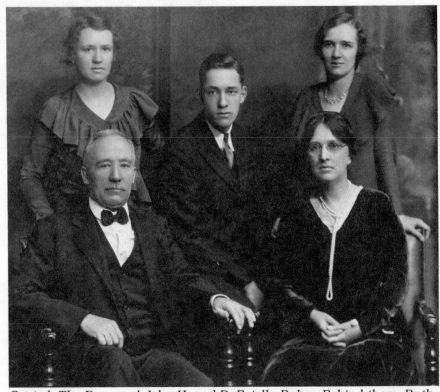

Seated: The Reverend John H. and D. Estella Raker. Behind them: Ruth, Conrad and Roberta Raker.

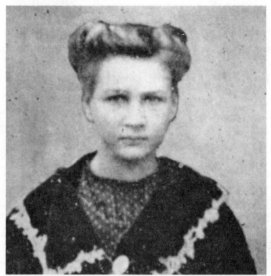

Viola Hunt, Good Shepherd's first resident, became the mother of twenty-three children.

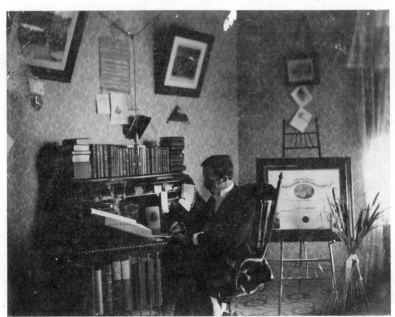

At this desk, in 1908, Papa Raker opened the letter asking him to find a home for a crippled orphan, Viola Hunt.

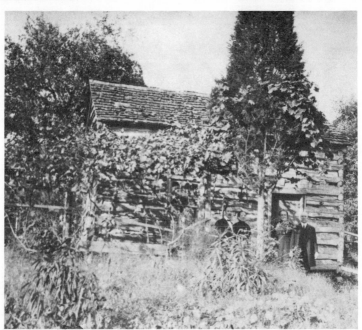

Standing in front of the log cabin in which he was born are Papa Raker; his sisters, Lydia Schlegel and Hattie Moyer and his brother, Fred D. Raker, M.D.

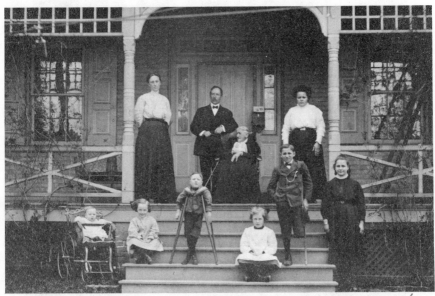

On the porch of the old farmhouse: Mama Raker, Papa Raker, Aunt Mary, unidentified girl. On the steps: Baby Sunshine, Roberta Raker, unidentified boy, Ruth Raker, Harold Bortz, Viola Hunt.

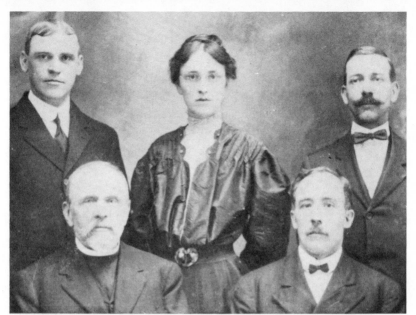

Good Shepherd's first board of trustees: The Rev. Ira W. Klick, secretary; the Rev. Prof. William Wackermagel, D.D., vice president; D. Estella Raker; the Rev. John H. Raker, president and superintendent; Robert W. Kurtz, treasurer, 1909.

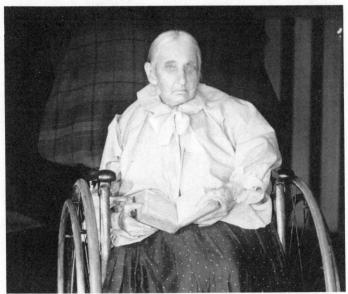

Aunt Polly Nauman entered The Good Shepherd Home when 105 years old and died when 108 years old in 1914.

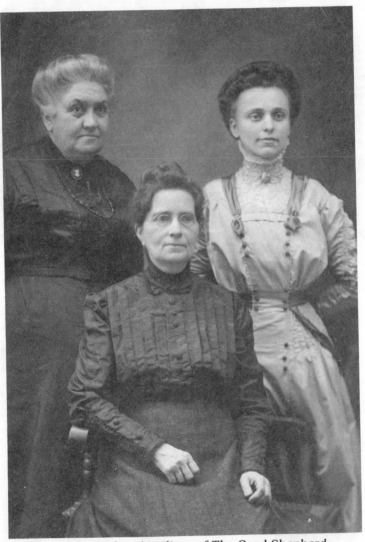

Officers of the Ladies Auxiliary of The Good Shepherd Home, 1909: Mrs. R.S. Diehl, treasurer; Miss Laura V. Keck, president; Mrs. Robert W. Kurtz, secretary.

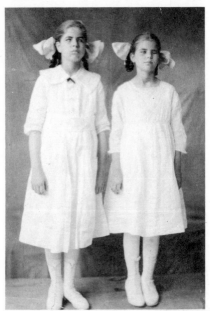

The blind sisters, Eva and Verna Pauley, 1919.

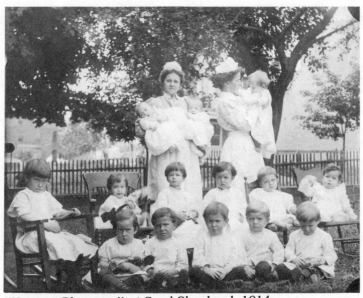

"Nursery Blossoms" at Good Shepherd, 1914.

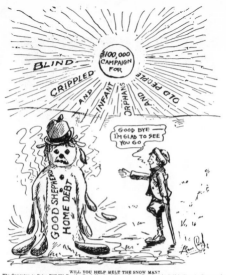

This Allentown Morning Call cartoon supporting the Good Shepherd Home's campaign to raise $100,000 in 1916 was drawn by Gene Carl, the first orphan boy to be accepted by The Orphan's Home in Topton, where Papa Raker had been superintendent.

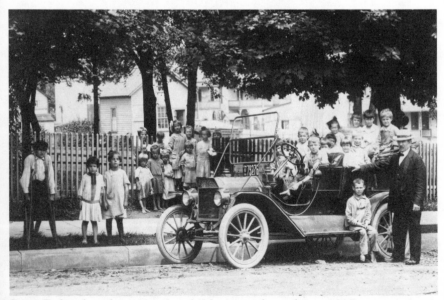

Papa Raker loved to take the children out for a drive, 1917.

A farm, a farm, my kingdom for a farm.

Sweet Charity
November-December 1914

Papa parodied Shakespeare's "King Richard III" in describing his dreams of a farm for The Good Shepherd Home. And he laid out just what farm he had in mind in that late 1914 issue of *Sweet Charity* and in the public press.

He had already gotten the support of the new advisory board in its first real action and that had translated into endorsement for the trustees—to the idea, at least.

There were two farms comprising 225 acres in what was then Salisbury Township—about a mile west and south of the Home. These were the holdings of the late attorney Marcus C.L. Kline, whose firm had handled the incorporation work for the Home.

"The Little Lehigh flows past the farms along their entire length and makes the northern boundary line of the farms," *The Morning Call* would describe the property. "On the south, they extend to the road that leads from the Emmaus road to the Salisbury Church.

"Most of the land lies on a plateau, level throughout to its greatest extent and rolling toward the stream.

"One of the farmhouses and the surrounding barns and other structures are along the road to the Trexler fisheries. All the buildings are in first-class condition."

Today, some of that land is part of Queen City Airport and some is the most beautiful section of

Allentown's park system, including the property where the Allentown Police Academy is located.

The Home got an option on the property in October 1914 by paying $50 down. The purchase price was $33,000. Of that amount, $1,000 had to be paid by January 1, 1915, and $12,000 on April 1. The Kline estate would take the rest on a 5 percent mortgage.

Because of problems of getting rid of the cattle on the properties, the Home was to get one farm of 145 acres on closing day and the other farm consisting of eighty acres on April 1, 1916.

This was a rather friendly transaction. The attorney handling things for the estate was Edwin K. Kline, the late Marcus's son and law partner. Edwin Kline was also the attorney for the Home.

Papa had long cherished the idea of a farm. It was to be part of his Great Plan.

The Home along St. John Street would remain the heart of everything. But the farms would eventually become a "Colony of Mercy," where a home would be built for epileptics. And a place at the New Jersey shore would provide a haven during the summer for those in Allentown.

Another objective was that the farms would give the able children and old people a chance for healthy employment, recreation and occasional change of environment.

The hired farm hands didn't have time to attend to a truck patch. So the Rev. Josiah S. Renninger, a retired Lutheran preacher in his late seventies, promised to oversee the truck patch and fruit trees. Pastor Renninger had been the founder or father of St. Luke's, St. Joseph's and Grace churches in Allentown.

By the time of his death in 1919, Rev. Renninger was instrumental in securing 1,500 fruit trees from friends for the farm. Many he carefully planted himself, saying he did not expect to eat of the fruit, but he did it for the crippled children and old people of the Home.

The first year of the farm, 400 grape vines, 100 peach trees, fifty apple trees and many raspberries and strawberries were planted. Also, cabbage, beans, peas, sweet corn, red beets and a lot of other vegetables.

Papa commented, "The boys have been doing most of the work under Rev. Renninger. If the patch reflects credit, the credit belongs to Rev. Renninger and the boys. If on the other hand the truck patch is no credit, the blame also belongs to them."

The strawberry patch at picking time became almost a shrine for the blind children. What would be repeated in *Sweet Charity* was a haunting picture of a boy with a crutch and two blind girls, the Pauley sisters, in that berry patch.

"Robert Burns could sit down and weep when he saw where the plow had separated the little mouse from its mother and destroyed its home," Papa wrote in cutlines under that picture.

"It was a pitiful sight, a touch of crippled helpless human nature, to see these blind children picking strawberries by touch, and it should make all the world akin and create a desire within us to help.

"If the immortal Burns could weep when he saw a little mouse had lost its mother and the little lamb that had broken its legs, what can and should not you and I do for these helpless ones that are created in our own image, the image of God.

"If such a scene does not move you, then your heart is dead and cold, fit for tragedy or treason. We have never seen a human being whose heart did not respond to such an appeal if the facts were clearly stated."

Yet another aim in acquiring the farms was that they could make money. Some people scoffed. But Dr. D.D. Fritch, the master farmer from Macungie, said they could be profitable.

Papa wanted a dairy herd so the children of the Home would have the best of fresh milk.

A few years earlier, the Home admitted two sick babies who were only a few weeks old. They became weaker and weaker.

One day, an attending physician said, "I am doing everything I can for these children, and I see your nurses are doing all they can, and yet the children do not thrive as they should. Suppose you have the milk analyzed and see if the children are getting the proper nourishment."

Tests subsequently showed the milk was skimmed and watered. Papa was stunned.

The two sick children died soon afterward in the hospital.

The man who supplied the milk secured it from a dozen different farmers. That left it in doubt: Just who took the cream out and who put the water in?

The Home changed milkmen, and Allentown afterwards fined the original supplier $50 for the same offense.

In recounting the incident, Papa said, "To succeed, we must be master of the situation. This is being accomplished by The Good Shepherd Home farms, where there will be no inducement for anyone to adulterate the milk. Here we know just what we are getting.

"Some claim milk from our farms would cost as much as if we bought it. We are confident it will not cost as much. But if it would cost more, we would be justified in our efforts to properly care for the children."

Papa raised the money for the January 1, 1915, payment of $1,000 but came up about $2,500 short on the $12,000 needed on closing day despite substantial newspaper coverage of the final countdown.

The sale was completed nonetheless. Papa got the $2,500 by giving his personal note to Lehigh Valley Trust Co.

That first day of ownership, he took some of the crippled children to the farms in his car. They greatly enjoyed it.

"The acquiring of the farms was a happy event at the Home," *The Morning Call* reported. "The achievement of Mr. Raker to secure the farms is considered a master stroke and one essential for the larger work of the Home."

And Papa was already using *The Call* to huckster for a horse. As the newspaper reported that April 3:

"There seems to be a great difficulty among the small boys in getting to and from the farm to the

Home, as there is no appropriate conveyance for them to travel with.

"What seems to be needed is an old horse, so the boys can take the many things necessary from the Home to the farm. At Topton, that same difficulty was experienced and the problem was ably solved when a resident donated a horse to the institution."

Within two weeks, he had six horses, including a span of fine iron grays worth $500 donated by Max Hess Sr., the department store proprietor. Hess wasn't in favor of the Home buying farms. He thought it would detract from the efforts at St. John Street, that it would spread the Rakers and their workers too thin. But once the Home committed itself to farming, Hess lent his help.

And so did a multitude of others.

Ten years earlier, while at Topton, Papa had given a bit of assistance to the local Mennonite Conference in setting up an orphans and old people's home at Center Valley, over the mountain south of Allentown. It excelled in farming and raising livestock.

Some Mennonites called Papa the father of that home. These brethren never forgot that kindness. They donated a Holstein bull calf to Good Shepherd farms. And in *Sweet Charity*, Papa included a paragraph on the calf's lineage and ancestral butterfat achievements, just as he'd give the lineage and academic achievements of some local dignitary.

Mennonites from a Sunday school in Center Valley also had another way of thanking The Good Shepherd Home. For a number of years, the Sunday school teachers and officers each Thanksgiving, Christmas and Easter visited Good Shepherd.

"They came before daylight and sang carols as only Mennonites who are used to singing in the open air can sing," Papa recalled. "They left a basket of fruit at each building and $5 at the main building and departed before we were able to be out and greet them. This was to show their love and respect for The Good Shepherd Home."

When the Mennonites sold their herd sometime later because they could no longer manage it, *Sweet*

Charity carried a story announcing the sale. It listed the production records of its top animals.

"Pregnant Thoughts" was a feature in *Sweet Charity* right from its opening issue. With the acquisition of the farmland, *Sweet Charity* sometimes had a second such feature, "Pregnant Farm Thoughts." And Papa used this column to hail the achievements, cite the needs and lament the failures of the farms.

* * *

A sample of 1915 Pregnant Farm Thoughts:

—The work on the farms consists of spraying potatoes, cultivating potatoes and corn, making hay and harvesting wheat.

—We started to raise black pigs. On the 16th of July, we got six little snow-white pigs.

—Some of the dark or discouraging things on the farm has been the fact that the crows and blackbirds pulled a great deal of our corn, and two little black pigs died.

—Some of our boys have been asking for permission to raise skunks on The Good Shepherd Home farms. We have no special or natural inclination for skunks, but we encourage every original idea any of our boys may have. The farms are especially for the children, and if our boys desire to raise skunks and will do the work, they shall have the opportunity.

—The Muhlenberg students are studying the social problems in a practical way. Tolstoy, the great Russian poet and philanthropist, said, "You can never properly feel for people unless you do the same kind of work which they do." To some of the students, it was their first corn-husking experience. The Home greatly appreciated the kindness. Thirteen additional helpers in a cornfield certainly helps.

—Our Thanksgiving dinner consisted of roosters from the farms, donated when they were small by the president of the Wilkes-Barre Conference, the Rev. Wilmer F. Heldt.

* * *

The children of the Home, girls and boys, had to pitch in to help the regular hired farmers. During the summer, the boys would work part of the day on the farm and spend part of it in a camp along the Little Lehigh. They lived in tents, leaky tents the first year, according to John Yost, who arrived at the Home in 1915.

When it came time for picking potatoes in the fall, Papa would go to the superintendent of schools and get the kids excused for a week or two.

And the Home paid the children for their work—ranging from a dime to a quarter a day, but pay nonetheless.

Farm ownership turned Papa into a militant farmer, too. He railed against government interference. He anguished over the high price of equipment compared with the low return for the crops.

Sometimes, too, he faced problems with bad help. Not only had one farm worker stolen some chickens, he had fed some of the Home boys booze before departing.

Papa had his farm causes, just like his causes for the crippled. Good cows' milk was fine for the children. Goats' milk was even better.

He had raised goats as a youngster back in Northumberland County. And he acquired some for the Home farms.

Papa expounded at length on the value of goat's milk in the May-June 1919 issue of *Sweet Charity*.

"We once read somewhere that the milk of the goat came nearest to human milk.

"Ten years ago, when we started to take sick infant motherless children, we were somewhat discouraged by the Rev. Dr. Hart, director of the Child Helping Department of the Russell Sage Foundation. He stated that statistics showed the mortality in children's homes was greater than in the slums from which they came.

"The doctor said, 'If The Good Shepherd Home can reduce the mortality, your reputation is made.'

"For over ten years, we have tried every conceivable method at the suggestion of our physicians and have

77

greatly reduced the mortality. But we also feel convinced that some of our children were carried to the cemetery plot who should be living today to bless and benefit the world.

"This is an awful assertion. We did the best we knew, but the trouble was we did not know enough."

Papa maintained that much tuberculosis in children came from tuberculosis in cows, transmitted through the milk.

"The ideal milk for the child is human milk from healthy unimpregnated mothers. Its only substitute is from matured healthy unimpregnated milch goats. The most noted authorities in Europe and America agree the qualities of goats milk lie in its immunity from the danger of carrying the germs of tuberculosis, making it the best of all foods.

"Mother's milk given from the bottle will not have as good results as when drinking direct from the breast.

"We are convinced that there is nothing that will prevent disease and restore health to the sick infant motherless child like goats milk direct from the goat.

"It is sad to think some people are so overly sensitive with respect to goats milk that they would sooner bury those they love than nurse them direct from a clean, healthy, life-giving goat.

"If our venture proves successful, as we believe it will, The Good Shepherd Home will secure a number of goats so we can give the best the world can give to the delicate, sick, motherless child. In extreme cases, we will nurse the child direct from the goat. We will do anything and everything we can to help our children."

And that issue of *Sweet Charity* carried a picture of a worker holding a child who was nursing from a goat.

* * *

Things went well with the farm until the city decided it wanted to take at least part of it for a park system along the Little Lehigh Creek.

This was one issue the public press and *Sweet Charity* saw in widely differing ways. The time was July 1925.

Gen. Harry C. Trexler—industrialist, owner of vast farmlands and philanthropist—was the leader in an effort to establish an Allentown city park along the course of the Little Lehigh Creek.

Sweet Charity preferred to label Trexler "one of the chief agitators" of this proposal.

The Morning Call that July 8 reported:

"The first definite step toward the creation of the Little Lehigh park was taken yesterday when Gen. Trexler, Col. Edward M. Young, John Leh for the Leh estate and E.N. Kroninger gave approximately 150 acres of ground without charge to the city.

"The donation by these progressive citizens was made at a meeting of the city planning commission, attended by other land owners whose property is in the area surveyed for the park which will be three and a half miles in length.

"On the hill crests on each bank of the river a drive is planned in a manner which will permit a beautiful panorama of the scenic splendors of the Little Lehigh Valley."

While only donations of land from the four were announced, the other owners whose property will be included in the park "manifested a spirit of cooperation and will do all in their power to make the park a reality through generous concessions to the city," *The Call* story contended.

It noted The Good Shepherd Home farm was along the stretch and also a farm Papa himself owned near Bogert's Bridge, a covered bridge that still survives.

Rev. Raker feels very kindly toward the subject and the matter will be placed before the trustees by the planning commission, the story said.

In some ways, Papa did feel kindly toward the park idea. He predicted in *Sweet Charity* that soon with the park and the boulevards around it, the area would rival in beauty and grandeur Wissahickon Drive in Fairmount Park in Philadelphia.

And he said that the most impressive sight on a drive through the park would be The Good Shepherd Colony of Mercy, that home for epileptics he kept talking about, on high ground overlooking the park—

79

acreage the city wasn't planning to take.

But those mentions about generous concessions in *The Call* just weren't so, as far as Papa was concerned.

As he told *Sweet Charity* readers, this was an issue between the clean, rich, expanding City of Allentown which just announced it had over $1 million in its treasury versus The Good Shepherd Home with an empty treasury and a deficit of over $10,000 in its maintenance fund.

"No one who knows the struggles and sacrifices of the Home would for one moment expect that the crippled, the blind, the epileptic and sickly orphan children and helpless, homeless old people should help to donate for this proposed park.

"The self-respecting citizens of Allentown would resent it. No one expects it.

"Some people say anything is good enough for the crippled and blind orphan child. Some even suggested the Home sell its valuable farms and locate somewhere where land is cheap."

Papa pointed out there was just as much wisdom in locating the park where land is cheap.

Somebody has to protect the crippled and the blind children, Papa said. The Home insists on doing this under the most favorable circumstances.

"If the Home had not insisted continually, it would have been pushed off the map long ago.

"Years ago, the Home realized it needed a few farms to carry out its great work in addition to the city plant. We asked the Lord's guidance and we believe were divinely directed.

"Those who were intimately connected with the appeal and the purchase understand it. Others cannot. The farms are just what the Home wanted and, above all, just what the Home needs.

"To sell at any price would be to underestimate our work and make us feel guilty of deserting our Lord's cause, like Judas of old."

So much for the "generous concessions" mythology of the local press.

If the land had to go, Papa felt obligated to get the top dollar.

In early 1926, The Good Shepherd trustees passed a resolution saying that while they favored the location of the proposed boulevard and other public improvements in our city, they felt as the trustees of a charitable institution that they hadn't the moral right to sell property acquired for the expansion of the Home through gifts from a wide circle of supporters and which was part of their plans to establish a colony of mercy.

"The boulevard, moreover, would take from our farms all the dwellings and outbuildings and would make the farming on which we depend for produce more expensive than at present."

It would be five more years before the city was to put its park plan into operation. Then, a board of viewers set the price at $24,000.

Papa lamented to the board, "$24,000 for 48 acres, two large barns, two large houses, one small house, two two-story summer houses and all buildings connected with the farms.

"What shall the Home do? What can the Home do?"

Papa had a contingency plan of sorts. He owned a farm himself just to the west in the area of Bogert's Bridge, the only surviving covered bridge in Allentown. The buildings on that land would serve the Home and, just before his death in 1941, Papa sold that farm to the Home.

Not all was gloom at the farm in that era.

An acre of potatoes for Good Shepherd had meant a lot to Papa even back before the Home had a farm.

In 1914, he had praised nine members of St. John's Lutheran Church in Quakertown for planting an acre of potatoes for the Home. "Let others follow this practical way to help the helpless. St. John's, Quakertown, is showing its faith in all lines of church work," he proclaimed in *Sweet Charity*.

But Papa had one of his proudest agricultural moments in 1931 when the farm joined the 400 Bushel Potato Club, raising 427 bushels on a measured acre. That was third among the ten Lehigh County farmers who were added to the club that year. And farmer Raker was already predicting the Home's farm would be in the 500 Bushel Club the next year.

Much of the credit belonged to Clayton Rosenberger, the superintendent of the farms, a Mennonite from the Spinnerstown area of Bucks County.

Papa commented, "Some time ago, we heard a discussion on the question: Which of the three religious denominations, Mennonite, Lutheran and Reformed, were the best farmers. The persons taking part in the discussion were all Lutheran and Reformed, and they decided the Mennonite Church had the best farmers."

* * *

In Connie Raker's era some devastating news about the farm began arriving in January 1943. Real estate broker Roscoe Jarrett asked the board to retain him in the expected upcoming dealings with the federal government.

Mack Motor Co. (now Mack Trucks) was to use its sprawling 5-C plant for building airplanes, supervised by Vultee Aircraft Corporation, Connie told the board.

"As you know, the 5-C plant is practically across the Emmaus Pike from the southeast boundary of our farm. They will take practically all the plateau land from the pike to the Little Lehigh Creek. This is to be used as an airfield."

The government didn't want to purchase the land, but to lease it for the duration. Lease or own, the government action would have a profound effect upon the Home's future farm program.

"It will leave us considerably less than one hundred acres, land on an incline, difficult for farming."

Real estate man Jarrett appeared at the next board session, explaining that the War Department was taking over 700 to 1,000 acres in and around the Good Shepherd farm. The board did the only thing left to do—name a committee that included Connie and Judge James F. Henninger, the board president, to negotiate with the government.

Good Shepherd had 320 acres under cultivation—270 acres of its own and fifty rented from Robert

Young. The government wanted 213 of Good Shepherd's 270.

"We certainly should have a hundred acres in order to raise fodder for our cattle and have enough room for truck farming," Connie protested.

The grim news was outlined in *The Morning Call* of March 23, 1943. The U.S. government had gotten federal court approval to take by eminent domain approximately 325 acres along the Emmaus highway and extending westward to the east branch of Little Lehigh Parkway.

The land would be used by Vultee to manufacture torpedo bombers for the U.S. Navy.

Of that 325 acres, 213 acres represented the best of The Good Shepherd Home farm. Seizure forced the Home out of farming after nearly thirty years.

The Second War Powers Act gave the government the right to take immediate possession. Working out compensation with Good Shepherd and the other fourteen landowners would come later.

A huge airfield would be built with runways 300 feet wide. The planes would be constructed at Mack's 5-C on the other side of the Emmaus highway and towed across the road to the airfield to be tested.

The newspaper story concluded:

"Thus, planes will be flying very soon over land for which its owners long have had carefully cherished plans of an entirely different order.

"The Good Shepherd Home farms lose 213 acres that, with nearby leased land that has also been condemned, had been tilled for a number of years to supply the inmates of the Home with food and provided light employment for a considerable number of the inmates during the open months of the year.

"It also takes the site which the Rev. Dr. John H. Raker had planned as a colony for epileptics—a plan he conceived almost thirty years ago and left to his son to carry out in his memory.

"It has been his idea to have a balanced institutional setup through construction of a Home in the city, one in the country and a third at a seashore point."

Connie reported to the board: "The serious blow has

been keenly felt, especially with regard to our proposed colony for epileptics. All the land that was dedicated for this purpose will serve as an airfield for torpedo bombers."

What remained were a house and barn just south of Bogert's Covered Bridge, an orchard of about fifteen acres, a little woodland and about eight acres to actually farm. The Home would eventually sell part of the orchard to attorney William Hudders, Connie's brother-in-law, and the rest to the city.

Meanwhile, the federal government offered Good Shepherd $575 an acre for much of the condemned land, $550 an acre for the rest. The board countered by asking for $800 an acre. When it learned others were getting up to $1,000 an acre, it upped its counter offer to that figure.

What the Home got was $121,475—the original price quoted by the government, plus about $12,000 in interest . . . more than a year later.

It invested the money in U.S. Treasury Bonds.

What the taxpayers got from Vultee was a fantastic failure. Some 504 planes were scheduled to be built by the end of 1944. Only two were built.

Not until 1945, with the end of the war approaching, did the plant turn out 178 more bombers. None ever made it into combat.

The Navy poured $85 million into the project. It came to something like $472,000 per plane while General Motors was building the same plane for $70,000.

An investigating Congressman called the project "a great job of bungling." The Navy blamed Vultee, and Vultee blamed the Navy. The local paper editorialized: "Never again probably will so many persons be thrown into so many jobs for which they are unfitted and ignorant and receive so much money for incompetency and ignorance."

By the fall of 1945, Mack was preparing to take back its 5-C plant, and General Electric Co. took over various buildings constructed during wartime to supplement the Mack facilities.

At about that time also, the Vultee people took

Connie and several members of the Home's "farm purchasing committee" over what once had been the farm.

They determined that considerably over half the original farm lay under runways and hangars. The property, even if it could be acquired, was unsuitable and unprofitable for Good Shepherd's use.

While Vultee was a short-term disaster, the property was eventually developed into Queen City Airport for use by smaller private and commercial planes.

*   *   *

In late 1945, The Good Shepherd Home went back into farming with the purchase of two adjoining properties totaling 180 acres along Route 222 at East Texas Road near the village of Wescosville, several miles west of Allentown. The price for the two was $18,000. The larger one, 140 acres owned by Allentown attorney Louis M. Stamberg, had a house and farm buildings. They would be renovated.

Truck farming and the raising of livestock would supply food for the Home, Connie announced. But the long-term purpose of the purchase was to fulfill his father's dream of a colony for epileptics.

Elam Smith and his wife, Arlene, of Kempton R. 1 were hired as the farm family to run the place. Master farmer Robert Aten of Macungie, a member of the board of trustees, was helping with advice.

Connie noted the trouble in the past of using raw milk. The new farm had aligned itself with the Lehigh Valley Cooperative Farmers. It would ship its milk to Lehigh Valley and then buy what pasteurized milk it needed from the co-op.

Good Shepherd went out of the farming business for good in 1960. It sold that Wescoesville property to the Shepherd Hills Farms Inc. represented by Allentown attorney Paul McGinley.

Connie told *Sweet Charity* readers:

"One of my father's fondest dreams was a colony of mercy for epileptics. For this, two farms were purchased, the idea being that epileptics needed a large land area to separate them from the rest of society. This was the traditional concept—that in a community of their own kind beneficial relaxation was achieved.

"New drugs have changed the idea completely. Though these drugs do not cure epilepsy, they minimize the violence of the attacks to such a degree that epileptics can now live quite comfortably with others."

Like other groups of supposedly handicapped or crippled, the epileptics had been mainstreamed.

The Wescosville farm became part of a development that we know today as Shepherd Hills. It joined Little Lehigh Parkway and Queen City Airport in what might be called The Good Shepherd Home Farms Alumni Association. ❖

Population—47 children, 9 old people: 15 crippled, 3 cannot walk even with crutches, 3 cannot speak, 1 cannot move, 27 were babies when brought in.

Sweet Charity
1914

Papa Raker was talking about a $100,000 campaign as early as 1912. Like so many other things he did, he warned people ahead of time that this campaign was coming. He talked through his dreams on the pages of *Sweet Charity*.

The September-October issue of 1912 carried this notation from the fourth anniversary celebration: "Labor Day marked the inauguration of plans to be formulated and perfected for the raising of a $100,000 fund with which to enlarge the Home and meet the crying need of the helpless crippled, blind and infant orphan."

But the drive would be postponed until the spring of 1916. And it would follow campaigns by just about every other major charity in the Allentown area within a six-month period in 1915.

The Allentown YMCA had started it off with a successful campaign for $120,000. Allentown College for Women (Cedar Crest) raised over $75,000 in a week's time. Sacred Heart Hospital with its tag day netted over $8,000 in a day and the Associated Charities got $6,000 in a three-day effort.

Then, Muhlenberg College, with a goal of $60,000, raised $68,000 within a week and could easily have raised more.

Yet, despite all this going before, Good Shepherd succeeded.

Papa called the Advisory Board together early in 1916. "It is the opportunity of a lifetime," Papa said. "If the campaign is properly managed, the needed amount to put the Home on a solid basis can be secured."

The Home had property worth $100,000—including the farms—set against a debt of $47,000.

The funds from the drive would be used to remove the debt, put a "respectable building" at the corner of Sixth and St. John and help enlarge the existing buildings on the city property.

With only one of the two farms available in the first year of farming, the Home raised 2,900 bushels of potatoes, 2,000 bushels of corn, 700 bushels of oats, 172 bushels of wheat and thirty tons of hay. Surely production would be doubled in 1915 with both farms in Good Shepherd's hands.

The Home was already extensively recognized. Money and other gifts had come from sixteen different states. Papa asked: Why shouldn't it? After all, the Home received needy ones from all denominations, even those whom other institutions refused to take.

Pennsylvania had 4,000 blind children. Yet Good Shepherd was the only institution to accept such children.

The Advisory Board concluded the goal of the campaign should be at least $100,000 "for this most worthy institution of God."

Papa ultimately took his question to the Highest Authority—his Lord.

He read passages of Scripture from Genesis, Psalms, Isaiah and Lamentations that Dr. Wackernagel suggested he read, including the words: "The Lord is good unto them that wait for Him, to the soul that seeketh him." He meditated in the silent watches of the night.

And he put it as straight to the Lord as he did to the Advisory Board.

"We asked the Lord the following questions: Lord, do You really want us to have this campaign? If You do not want it, we don't want it either.

"Is this campaign for the glory of God and helpless humanity?

"Have we been sufficiently humbled in our work at The Good Shepherd Home to seek only Thy favor, Thy will, and have we the burning desire needed to help the needy ones in our Home and the cold, half-clad, suffering ones who are constantly knocking at our doors?"

Papa concluded, "We believe the Lord answers all these questions in the affirmative. We believe the Lord is beckoning you and me to help in The Good Shepherd Home campaign.

"Let us show our faith by our works."

Papa pointed out that he had stood practically alone as a solicitor in the early months of 1915 in securing the $13,000 needed as the down payment for the farms.

Here, in this $100,000 campaign, there were several hundred people who would help with a "united, organized, well-tried plan, with all the newspapers of the city and the eastern part of the state eager, willing and enthusiastic to help one of the most worthy institutions in the country."

He had already lined up David A. Miller, the owner of *The Morning Call* in Allentown, to head up the publicity committee for the drive and Eugene Carl, now a cartoonist for the paper, to create drawings to illustrate the needs of the campaign once it was underway. That was the same Gene Carl who had done the art work for the front cover of *Sweet Charity* in its first years, the first orphan from the Topton Home. Papa was one to go back again and again to those who helped him in earlier years and find them willing to help once more.

He sent a personal letter to all ministers in the area asking them—"if it is not contrary to your custom"—to announce the campaign in their churches. It would run from April 25 to May 3.

"It is not contrary to the custom of the Home to receive the most needy children and old people of all denominations.

"We hope and pray that your church will never be in need of a home for a crippled, blind or sickly child or old person. But if in the Providence of God this should happen, the sheltering arms of The Good Shepherd Home will be extended to you as far as we possibly can."

He published 40,000 copies of the April-May *Sweet Charity* to coincide with the campaign. The cover was a Carl drawing of a barefoot crippled girl apparently sobbing against the front of what had been her home—where there is a black crepe posted on the door and next to it a sign, "Room to Let."

The heading under it said: THE UNOBSERVED HUMAN TRAGEDY OF THE BROKEN HOME AND THE CRIPPLED CHILD.

The picture is not drawn on the imagination or fancy of the human brain, *Sweet Charity* said. Rather, it deals with the everyday cold realities of life facing those who seek help from The Good Shepherd Home.

Papa and Wilson Arbogast, the Allentown meat packer, volunteered for the executive committee that would head the drive. But Papa was absolutely shameless in his tactics for enlisting the six others he figured he needed for that executive committee.

He and Arbogast tried three times in vain to get a yes from Dr. Robert B. Klotz, a real estate man who had a prominent part in a drive recently concluded for Muhlenberg College. Klotz had too much business on his hands, a building boom in fact, and a multitude of physical ills.

Papa said he had already prayed over this and had the assurance that the Lord wanted Klotz on the executive committee. But, as Papa observed, Klotz hadn't gotten the word. It came later.

Just to get rid of Papa and Arbogast, Klotz said he'd

show up at the organizing meeting of the drive's executive committee. And as a man of his word, he did.

At the meeting, the student deacon brought ten crippled boys to the office where the men gathered. One boy, a bright-faced lad, was carried and laid on his stomach on the floor. This youngster, paralyzed in both legs and one arm, tried to work his way toward Klotz.

The man, moved with compassion, asked the boy how he was. The lad answered with a smile, "I am all right."

Papa would say later, that was the moment when the Lord communicated to Klotz that he was to be a member of the executive committee.

The others in the group were Harvey E. Bohner, proprietor of a downtown furniture house; Elmer Heimbach, who previously ran a successful $75,000 campaign for Allentown College for Women (now Cedar Crest); Herbert W. Elvidge, secretary of the Allentown YMCA and perhaps the one most skilled in running campaigns in the Lehigh Valley; F.P. McDermott, head of an engineering company; and Phaon Diehl, founder of a furniture house.

They all turned to Arbogast as chairman, a man Papa described as "firm in purpose, gentle in execution, justly confident in his own judgment, yet generously open to the opinions of others" and, by Arbogast's own admission, no orator.

Neither was Moses, Papa reminded. And the Lord appointed Aaron to do the speaking for him.

Well, Providence was at work here, too, just as in those Old Testament days. The committee had its own Aaron, the silver-tongued Harvey E. Bohner "who conducted that part of the campaign in a most pleasing and acceptable manner, keeping the teams in good humor with an enthusiasm that was contagious."

Two hundred people attended the kickoff meeting. It opened with Scripture and a prayer—given by Dr. Wackernagel. That seemed to be the way Papa ran any venture. His own last testament and will began with a prayer.

91

There was even a campaign poet, real estate man Gilbert H. Aymar, the individual who taught Helen Keller how to operate a typewriter.

All denominations were represented. Good feeling prevailed.

Sixteen teams—four of them comprised entirely of women—were to handle the solicitation of several thousand names.

And the first three days of the effort, the solicitors were besieged by rain.

The final day came with $30,000 still needed.

Florist Edward N. Kroninger secured the free service of thirty automobiles with chauffeurs to take canvassers to see the people. Three reports were given that day—one at noon, another at 6 p.m. and another at 9.

At this last meeting, over $95,000 was reported with a number of indefinite promises and at least a third of the people not seen.

The Bible says Joshua once stopped the sun to finish his task. The captains and lieutenants of the campaign teams were confident that all they needed was a little more time. So they underwrote the amount necessary to reach the $100,000.

They would prove to be right. With some additional time, they got the pledged total just over that $100,000 goal.

The achievement came despite rumors that had plagued Papa for years—that the Home was a stock company and the stock owned by a few men and that the deeds were in the names of a few men. "You fight me with rumors," Papa said in quoting Cicero.

To deal with this, he had the charter, bylaws, constitution and the ten deeds of the Home placed in the offices of a downtown furniture store for all to inspect.

The cash initially given was sizable compared with those other recent drives in Allentown. But the pledges were for two years, with the first money not due until 1917. And like pledges for anything, some of the promised money never did come in.

What was amazing about this campaign was that it

involved more people than all the other six campaigns that preceded it combined. The average gift was smaller, but the interest wider.

It advertised Good Shepherd beyond all calculation. And it blessed those who worked in the campaign and those who responded.

"The community is elevated to an extent no one can measure," Papa said.

It would be about fifty years before the Home would again go to a public drive for funds.

There were plenty of needs in the decades in between, sometimes crying needs in the Depression years when forty or fifty people would knock on Good Shepherd's door on a Sunday for a meal—over and above its own residents and workers and their families to feed.

But the gifts and bequests of those whose hearts were touched by the Home sustained the daily operation. And when major projects came along, they were backed by the quiet asking of friends for special help. ❖

What a pleasure to work in Christ's cause in an age like ours.

Sweet Charity
November-December 1915

There's a multitude of other things that should be touched upon from those early years of the Home. They bear no particular pattern except they span the silly to the serious in a Home that seemed to experience almost everything.

Surely this history of the Home should note that one of the first things done by Harry Filer, a youngster on crutches who became Good Shepherd's first graduate of Allentown High, on his very first day was to put firecrackers in Papa Raker's hat.

Further, Papa said the best potato picker at the farm was the most mischievous boy at the Home. And that was apparently someone other than Harry.

Papa advised *Sweet Charity* readers:

"Some of our friends say they could not visit The Good Shepherd Home because they were too tender-hearted and would be too much affected by seeing the crippled and blind children at the Home. If these tender-hearted people would visit the Home long enough to see some of our overly active or naughty crippled boys, they would soon change their minds.

"The crippled boys are just like other boys."

And there's the story of Grandma Weiser, Mama Raker's mother, who served for long periods of time as the cook in the early years of the Home. She even was on the payroll for a while in that capacity.

Mama Raker, for all her sainted virtues, was a terrible cook. And the Home had trouble keeping cooks. So Grandma Weiser would fill in until new help was secured and then she'd return home to Lebanon.

Randolph Kulp, a St. John Street neighbor, says that when he was a youngster, Connie Raker would drop in at his home some evenings and sometimes would stay for a meal. On one such visit, Connie told the Kulps this incident:

Papa and Mama got into a tiff on one occasion and she threatened to go home to mother. Papa chimed in, "Good, I'll go along with you. That way I'll get a decent meal."

A serious fire at the Home in 1910 had its light aftermath.

On a Sunday in July, a six-year-old crippled orphan boy at the Home noticed boys in the street playing with matches and firecrackers. Toward evening, he took some matches and lit paper in a small annex west of the main building that was used for tools and old clothing. The fire smoldered until the children and old people retired for the night at about 8 o'clock.

A nurse had gone to church. Papa was in East Allentown in a pulpit exchange, serving Communion. Mama was sitting on the east side of the building with her friend from Lebanon, Hattie Coover, who was visiting.

"Fire! Fire! The Good Shepherd Home is on fire," a neighbor yelled.

Neighbors helped bring the children and old people out of the building. Mama herself brought two of the little ones down from the second floor as well as Aunt Mary Eisenhard.

Fireman Willis Daubenspeck of the nearby Fairview Co. proved the real hero. He dashed through smoke and flames up two flights of stairs to rescue a little child still on the third floor.

No one was hurt. Some furniture, including an organ, was destroyed. So was Aunt Mary's memorial certificate of twenty-five years as superintendent of St.

Michael's Sunday School. Most of the damage to the building and the furniture was covered by insurance.

All of Papa's sermons were also destroyed—eighteen years of diligent work reduced to ashes. He tried to comfort himself with the thought that the fire insurance company would make a liberal allowance for his great loss. But the insurance company would not allow a cent for what had been over 1,000 sermons.

"Corporations are said to have no souls," Papa said in 1910. "Thus, they would not be able to appreciate the value of a sermon."

He shared his misfortune with some of his closest brethren in the ministry, expecting their sympathy. Instead, they snickered. One said, "It was a blessing in disguise."

The first Lutheran minister admitted into the Home was an exceedingly pious, God-fearing man. He did not concern himself about earthly possessions, and it was taken for granted that he had some money when he entered the Home. Nothing, however, was mentioned about it.

One day, he asked Papa if he could have the percentage the Home allowed designated agents for new subscribers to *Sweet Charity*, half the fifty-cent subscription price. Papa said he was welcome to it. But it raised Papa's suspicions that the old preacher was short financially.

In his last illness, the preacher asked for ice cream. A nurse said she thought he should pay for such things himself. Papa told her to get the man what he wanted without asking questions about it.

"We were with him in his last hour," Papa said. "It was no ordinary occasion. The room was filled with heavenly electricity.

"After a subdued silence and a short prayer, we gathered his belongings together and put the more important things in his trunk. To our surprise and chagrin, we found this man of God did not have one penny in his pocket or in his name."

Surely, there were some little things this man longed for that he would have requested if he had some money in his name. It was a shame to let this man die without a penny when the Lord had blessed and prospered the Home, Papa told the board of trustees. And the board approved a fund to provide the old people who were without funds with fifty cents a month for spending money and some also for the children for offering for church and Sunday school.

Papa more than once told of a lesson learned from an aged janitor at the Topton Home that proved helpful in dealing with the old people at Good Shepherd.

This worker was a religious man and exceedingly kind to the children. But if he didn't get to see his former home for three or four months, he became so irritable it was almost impossible to deal with him. Once, in such a mood, he struck one of the boys with a piece of iron a blow that might have been fatal.

By accident, Papa found that by sending this janitor back near his old home when he got this homesick feeling, the man would soon return cheerful and happy.

It's that way with most old people, Papa observed. They seem to forget at times that things are not what they used to be. They imagine that at the old homestead everything was as it used to be in the happiest days of their lives.

"We have often heard visitors say to our guests: 'If I had a good home like this, where I had enough to eat and a good warm bed to sleep, clothing to wear, papers and good books to read, medicine, doctor and minister provided, I would be satisfied and not want to leave my room.'

"Just try such a person for a short time and you will soon hear a different story," Papa said.

So when the old people became dissatisfied or homesick or cranky, Papa found the best thing was to put them in the automobile and, if possible, take them to the scenes of their childhood or former home, and bring them back from their bumpy ride with different ideas, happy and contented.

The same thing works wonders with the help, Papa said.

"We have spent whole days taking the old people

and children to the strawberry patches on the farms, and they are now classed among our happiest days, and their happiness increases with age."

Mama was the first member of the original board to be replaced. She left in September 1915, to be succeeded by meat packer Wilson Arbogast, the man who led the successful $100,000 campaign.

The board minutes for that meeting report: "In view of the fact that Supt. and Mrs. Raker recognized the desirability of having an experienced businessman as a member of the board of trustees, Mrs. Raker volunteered to resign to make room for such a man."

Arbogast was president of Arbogast and Bastian, a former member of City Council and a vice president of the first citywide school board.

He had supplied the Home with over $500 worth of meat a year for a number of years. He taught school for a year in the mid-1870s back in Mahanoy Township of Northumberland County where Papa grew up. He was a member of St. John's Lutheran Church in Allentown.

Because he was sick, Arbogast missed the victory dinner that he helped sponsor for the completion of the $100,000 drive in 1915. And he continued to be plagued by illness and often was absent from meetings once he was named to the board. He died in 1924 after a protracted illness.

Mama lived until 1963, though she never returned to the board. She was the first of what were only two women who would serve on the board over its first sixty years.

Almost from the beginning, there were rumblings within the Evangelical Lutheran Ministerium of Pennsylvania for representation on the board.

In the spring of 1910, the Home first approached the synod president for recognition and a visiting committee like the Topton Orphanage and other Lutheran homes within the territory whose trustees were not elected by the Ministerium.

Before people asked, Papa himself raised the question: Why go to the Ministerium in the first place if it would not help in founding the Home?

Papa answered that he was a Lutheran home missionary and it was as natural for him to look to his church as it was for a child to look to its mother.

Further, all board members were staunch Lutherans, and this gave the Home another tilt in that direction.

Finally, the Lutheranism of the Home was so Christ-like, so much like the Good Samaritan, that it was not objectionable, but sweet and attractive to the general public.

Synod took the approach that by having its visiting group, it was both serving as a watchdog and imparting its blessing on the Home.

And that fall, in speaking at the Home's second Anniversary Day, Synod President E. T. Horn assured the audience that the Ministerium would guard over the management of the Home to make sure their confidence in it was not misplaced.

In 1916, a synod committee recommended The Good Shepherd Board of Trustees be increased. It sent five representatives to meet with the Home's board about this.

Like Joseph of old showing his father all the glories of Egypt, the board tried to show the special committee all the glorious prospects of the Home. It made arrangements to take the committee members over all the buildings and farms. But the visitors couldn't spare the time.

The Home, however, did say it already intended to increase the size of the board to seven, perhaps even to nine.

The synod people asked that some of those members be chosen by the Ministerium or its Allentown Conference. And they admitted this was to try to satisfy a small dissatisfied element in synod.

Papa told them that this small element never did anything for the Home, constantly worked against it and, further, showed no signs of repentance. Placate that bunch and you anger the vast host of friends who have been liberal, loyal and faithful to the cause of Good Shepherd.

The Good Shepherd trustees said: We're willing to change if we can be shown that some other way is better than our own. But we hesitate to embrace a program not found working successfully in any other institution. Let's just continue this business of having a visiting committee from synod.

The synod people went back to the Ministerium praising the Home and the Rakers to the utmost. Their recommendation was "that there be no relationship between the two bodies, formal or otherwise, except a mutual feeling of appreciation and goodwill."

What an uproar over that one sentence!

Papa expounded in *Sweet Charity*:

"Legally speaking, there may not be that close relationship between the two bodies. But the Home, as well as the Ministerium, is not under the law, but under the Gospel. As such, we claim a close relationship.

"We claim the Lutheran Church to be the mother of The Good Shepherd Home, and we want this faithful mother of ours to have full credit for what her child of faith has already done and for the great things it promises to do in the future.

"The time is coming when the Ministerium of Pennsylvania will be proud of The Good Shepherd Home.

"The Home serves the interests of the Ministerium . . . by taking care of the most helpless children of the Church, also the faithful homeless old people of our Church . . . .also our aged and disabled ministers of the Ministerium, who are not yet helped by the proposed pension fund, and tries to give them a glorious twilight while they live and a Christian burial when they die.

"Does this look as if there was no relationship between the two bodies?"

A special synod session in early 1917 got the report of its investigating committee, and that generated two hours of discussion. President Horn ruled that if the "no relationship" statement was to stand, then no visiting committee would be sent by synod.

Speaker after speaker defended the Home. Some wanted to know why the Ministerium would now discriminate against Good Shepherd by withdrawing a visiting committee after having sent one for seven years.

It was finally and almost unanimously resolved "that it would be unwise to make any change, at this time, in the method of the management of The Good Shepherd Home or of the relationship of the Ministerium to it."

Good Shepherd did increase its board to seven later that year "to make it more representative" with the addition of Dr. Robert B. Klotz, the real estate man who had been on the executive committee of the $100,000 drive, and Dr. George Gebert, pastor of Zion Lutheran Church in Tamaqua.

And in 1921, the Home deferred somewhat by permitting one of its seven board members to be chosen by the Ministerium.

Synod's choice by unanimous vote was Dr. Solomon E. Ochsenford, pastor of St. John's Lutheran in Bath and a member of the Home's Advisory Board since its inception.

Papa put Dr. Ochsenford's picture on the cover of the next issue of *Sweet Charity* and commented in the lead story on him inside: "Synod made a wise selection and the board of trustees received a congenial addition."

It almost sounded like Papa was mellowing.

The Great War, what we now call World War I, touched the Home in a variety of ways.

Papa predicted in the 1913 Christmas edition of *Sweet Charity* that President Wilson and Secretary of State William Jennings Bryan would not lead America into war.

But on the magazine's cover of January-February 1916, he showed a photo of five boys playing in the snow with a toy cannon and other wooden weaponry. The heading was: Preparedness at The Good Shepherd Home.

The cutlines under the picture said:

"As followers of the Prince of Peace, we are strong advocates of peace. The great aim of The Good Shepherd Home is to help the crippled and as far as possible prevent the making of cripples.

"We hear so much about preparedness for war that even the crippled orphan children unconsciously, like President Wilson, imbibe the imaginary spirit of war.

"You will notice that the chief advocates of PREPAREDNESS at The Good Shepherd Home, like at other places, are largely those who would not be expected to go to the front if a crisis arose. Observe the fort, cannon and flag on The Good Shepherd Home lawn."

And at the start of 1917, he told *Sweet Charity* readers he thought Christianity had so asserted itself that a war like the present one was impossible in the twentieth century.

"The warring countries are now calling for the boys, the young boys. Lord have mercy."

And he cited federal figures from the Civil War: Of the 5,175,484 "men" who enlisted, 4,494,276 were under twenty-one at the time of enlistment. More than 1,100,000 were under seventeen and over 100,000 were under fifteen. Only 63,000 were over age twenty-five.

"It is as bad as the slaughter of the innocents when the Saviour was born," Papa lamented. "Lord, make every nation sick of war."

But later in the same issue, he would add: "The Good Shepherd Home is against war, but the Home will do its utmost to care for the war orphans in case the need should arise."

By then, the Home had already taken in one child whose mother was dead and whose father was in the Italian army. Mama Raker would head the neighborhood unit of the Red Cross.

And Papa would put a service flag in the window of the main building and on the cover of the September-October 1917 *Sweet Charity* for Home boy Charles Schander, sixteen, who enlisted in the Medical Department. That issue carried three letters from Schander, including his talk of machine guns and trenches.

The January-February 1918 cover had two stars—for Schander and for Home worker Frank Herr, who enlisted in the ambulance service. "If Uncle Sam knew how much we needed Frank Herr to take care of our crippled boys, he would not have taken him from us," *Sweet Charity* said.

A coal shortage in January 1918 hit the Home so severely that Papa had the farmers cutting down the dead trees in the grove on the farm—to have the wood ready once the coal became exhausted.

Even people whose cities and towns were underlaid with coal suffered for want of fuel. The Good Shepherd Home was no exception. All Allentown was uneasy.

That January 30, *The Philadelphia Press* ran a large picture of crippled children from Good Shepherd and stated the Home was without coal and without funds to buy it. The paper also said the Home kept the children in bed to keep them from freezing.

"The fact is we were almost without coal in zero weather," Papa said. "The suffering, however, was only mentally."

Allentown Mayor Alfred L. Reichenbach saw the article and phoned the Home to set up a meeting with the local fuel administrator. A friend from Reading sent $100 to the mayor to buy coal for the Home.

Papa told the mayor the Home had paid its coal bills to January 1 and the Home's credit was good.

The fuel administrator made arrangements with the coal dealer nearest the Home to reserve a certain amount from each car for Good Shepherd.

Just then the Home received word that a large car of coal from the Wilkes-Barre Conference Centurion Band, headed by Rev. Paul Kunzman, had arrived. Teams from the farm hauled the coal to the Home in one day. ❖

The Good Shepherd has always had enough of the discouraging to keep us humble.

Sweet Charity
January-February 1921

The Lehigh County Medical Society in rather blunt terms told The Good Shepherd Home in 1920 to get out of town.

It hadn't been the first group or individual to make the suggestion that the Home abandon its quarters on Allentown's south side and move to its farm property a mile or so to the southwest, just outside the city limits.

The Rev. Jeremiah H. Ritter, a solicitor for the Home, had proposed the idea in 1915 within weeks after the Home acquired the farms. As the board minutes of June 16, 1915, show: "It was moved that the proposition of Rev. Ritter with reference to moving The Good Shepherd Home to the farms be deferred for future action."

Ritter apparently persisted. The board at its January 1917 meeting tabled another letter from Rev. Ritter about the relocation of the Home.

Yet, only two months later, the board appointed its entire membership as a committee "to look into the matter of a possible new and better location for the future home of this institution."

What made the Medical Society proposal different is

that it was done publicly and with the intent of enlisting other organizations to its stance.

And here as the Home's eightieth anniversary approaches, that firestorm still seems to have some burning embers. It brings renewed flame to Connie Raker's face when it's mentioned. Further, twice the Medical Society was asked for information on its records of the dispute. Nothing was forthcoming.

At the very start of 1920, the Home announced it was going after $150,000 for a new administration building at Sixth and St. John streets.

The one planned from the proceeds of the $100,000 drive of 1916 never came about. Some of the money went to pay off the mortgage on the farms and debts on other buildings. Some went for small immediate projects. Some pledged money just never did come in.

And with the war and its shortages, the cost of construction had gone up considerably.

With the announcement of what was obviously the intent of the Home to stay where it was, the Medical Society members at their annual gathering "for hygienic and economic reasons do urge and implore the Rev. John Raker and his worthy Board of Trustees to locate this Great Humanitarian Institution on the beautiful Good Shepherd Home farms instead of the present location in the city."

There was, of course, a certain amount of buttering up of the Home in the opening paragraphs of the resolution.

It lauded the Home as a "worthy and deserving charitable institution" located in Allentown's Twelfth Ward.

It pointed to a ten-column article in *The Morning Call* of the day before that outlined the $150,000 campaign. It cited figures from that article—property worth $140,000 with debts of only $12,000 and the two farms covering more than 200 acres on the beautiful banks of the Little Lehigh.

Then, it turned to the Home's property on St. John Street, a frontage of 480 feet with a depth of 170. "This site will in the near future be too small to accommodate all the buildings necessary for the rapidly growing institution."

The next three "whereas" paragraphs bespoke of the society's supposed concern:

—"Elderly people will the more comfortably spend their declining years in a quiet country home away from the dust, smoke, noise, excitement and vitiated atmosphere of a closely built up city section."

—"The poor, innocent and crippled children will be happier, thrive better and respond more promptly to the proper hygienic, medical and surgical treatments if allowed to roam freely on God's green earth, instead of being penned in by brick walls or compelled to play on concrete sidewalks or on traffic-laden and danger-beset city streets."

—"In consideration of the present values of real estate, the sale of the property held by the Home within the city limits would net such a snug sum that it would defray at least half the cost of the proposed new administration building."

The resolution passed unanimously. The printed copy of it that went to Papa and the board carried the signatures of Dr. Frederick R. Bausch, the Medical Society president, and Dr. W.F. Herbst, its secretary.

Further, copies were sent to the Allentown Planning Commission, city and county officials, the Chamber of Commerce, Federation of Churches, Rotary, Kiwanis, the daily papers "and all benevolent and beneficial organizations in the community."

In addition, the letter to Papa and the Home that accompanied the resolution said it came in a "spirit animated by the desire to do the most good for your worthy institution and for your wards."

The Bausch letter also claimed that "public sentiment freely condemns the present location of the institution as utterly unsuitable and entirely inadequate."

The afternoon *Chronicle & News* carried nothing on the proposal. *The Morning Call* played the story on a back page.

A week later, *The Evening Item* ran an editorial that remouthed the claims made by the Medical Society, hailed the worthiness of the Home, noted many of its supporters came from beyond the Allentown area, cited the Home's need for better quarters . . . and then avoided taking a stand on which location.

It correctly concluded, however: "Whatever move is decided upon will fix the location of the institution for years to come."

The Good Shepherd Home had been a member of the Chamber of Commerce since 1916. But that was apparently no deterrent for the Chamber's board of governors subsequently to endorse the Medical Society proposal. That was done at a February session that included Gen. Harry Clay Trexler and Col. Edward M. Young, two of the most powerful men in the community.

Allentown Rotary also devoted considerable discussion to the matter, in response to a copy of the Medical Society letter.

Dr. C.O. Henry said the inmates of the Home should not be "exhibited" with the idea of moving visitors to pity or charitable impulses.

Lehigh County Judge Clinton A. Groman said he strongly supported the erection of buildings on the Home farm where the children could get the benefit of the open air and the kind of life needed in treating their ills.

But newspaper proprietor David A. Miller, a member of the Home's advisory board, preached restraint. Get more information on the subject and also the opinion of Superintendent Raker and the trustees before rendering a decision, Miller urged.

Rotary seemed to take Miller's advice. It adopted a resolution to have a committee of Rotary meet with the Home's trustees on the question of moving Good Shepherd.

Papa and the trustees had an answer:

We're going ahead with our administration building at Sixth and St. John as we had planned.

Our eventual Great Plan of city, country and seashore is to have facilities on the farm and at the New Jersey shore as well as in Allentown. The farm, perhaps, may be the major location, particularly for a colony of mercy for epileptics.

In both the daily press and in *Sweet Charity*, Papa and the trustees took the position that the Medical Society did what it did because it only had one side of the story. And he told the doctors and the public that "when you hear our side, you'll be with us."

He cited the early hardships, the basic fact that no one else was willing to take the crippled and the infants.

"We spent eight years in two small rooms with wife and three children while the other part of the house was filled with crippled and blind children, old people and sick babies. We worked here for three and one-half years without a cent of salary. We bought a Ford touring car, used it almost exclusively for the Home and paid for the running expenses the first year.

"This was the sacrifice someone had to make to bring The Good Shepherd Home into existence."

He said city and country locations each had their advantages and disadvantages.

Generally, the Home's crippled boys are not suited to become farmers. Their defects are against them.

Some people forget that God's green earth isn't green in the winter in Lehigh County and that the Little Lehigh is too cold for bathing at that time of the year.

One great advantage of a Home in the city is that the children can attend Allentown's public schools.

"The public school is a great mixer and teaches many things not on the regular program," the board said. "For many of our children, the city schools are the ideal thing and cannot be duplicated on the farms.

"The public school is also a great saving to the Home, but the Home will not look upon expense or economies when it can help the child.

"The church and Sunday school as they will find them in life, the city library, the YMCA swimming pool in winter and the constant touch of contact with the best people are of infinite value to a boy or girl who has the ability for an education and whose soul longs for the higher things in life."

Papa and the board hit right at the sympathy question raised by Dr. Henry at Rotary.

The fact that people can easily get to the Home is another great advantage. And if the Home had started in the country, it wouldn't be a tenth of what it is today, the board said.

After all, the Good Samaritan had to see the man who fell among thieves to know to help him. And 5,000 prospective Good Samaritans were passing The Good Shepherd Home every day.

Papa, of course, had a story to illustrate.

Several years back, a lady from Quakertown attended the anniversary at Bethany Orphans' Home at Womelsdorf. While going home on the trolley and passing Good Shepherd, she saw a number of crippled boys on crutches. She was impressed with the sight.

She wrote, asking about the Home. Papa mailed her a copy of *Sweet Charity*.

The upshot was she sent donations, visited and enlisted the support of her friends, who also gave donations.

The trustees conceded a Home in the country has many advantages.

"To come in close touch with nature, with the birds and flowers, the fields and animal and vegetable life is of infinite value to a child. A great educator once said that chores on a farm were the best course in manual training."

The statement said the Home didn't underestimate the value of a place in the country.

But just buying the farms had been a sore point with many of the Home's friends. They simply opposed it as acquiring an unprofitable burden. They wanted Papa and the board to fix up the Home in the city and be satisfied.

A place at the seashore has special advantages for children who could be helped only by the sea air. It could also be a place where the helpers could recuperate. And if the crippled and sick are to be properly cared for, consideration has to be given to the helpers.

Papa had purchased two lots at Wildwood, N.J., before acquiring the first property in Allentown. But a new railroad had spoiled them for what he intended.

Nonetheless, something would be worked out eventually for a seashore resort.

"People who have money go to the seashore," Papa said. "When they see the special efforts The Good Shepherd Home is making to help the helpless children, it will repay the Home a hundredfold."

Papa said the Great Plan of city, country and seashore had been explained to some hesitant friends who at first had doubts about the plan. Once they had it explained to them, they were glad to give toward the $150,000 goal.

"It is the great cause and workable plan that appeal to men and women to give liberally and to remember the Home in their wills," Papa said. "Great things are in store for The Good Shepherd Home if it remains faithful to its sacred trust.

"The unique plan of city, country and seashore appeals to men of large vision and great enterprise . . . and correspondingly large donations and bequests follow."

Now, how could anyone still say no to that? Why, it would be positively indecent to ask Good Shepherd to break its sacred trust.

Time would show that the Colony of Mercy idea would be abandoned, despite Papa's prayers at what to him became sacred ground on a high spot on the farm that he had chosen for that colony.

The ultimate and joyous reason would come nearly forty years later. The treatment of epileptics had so advanced that there was no need for a separate place for them. Medication and other developments had put what once had been outcasts now fully and capably in society.

Time would also see the disappearance of the farm— after years of faithful service.

One part of it would be taken by eminent domain by Allentown in the mid-1920s for perhaps the most beautiful part of its park system. But before that, for perhaps a decade, Good Shepherd boys and girls had enjoyed summer camp along the banks of the Little Lehigh and held afternoon rehearsals for their band after working earlier in the day on the Home farm.

The rest of the farm would go in World War II, seized

110

by the Navy for a Vultee plant to manufacture fighter planes and an airstrip to send them on their way. This would be a magnificent government failure.

Yes, there was another Good Shepherd Home farm purchased in Wescosville, a village west of Allentown at a time—1945— when villages around Allentown could still be clearly defined. It was put into spanking fine shape, joined the local milk cooperative and served the Home well until it was sold in 1960.

The seashore idea simply never came about. There had been opposition by nearby property owners when Papa had looked at some possibilities at the Jersey shore.

Those developments are parts of bits and pieces of other chapters.

What was more immediate was that Papa found an angel for that new main building. His name was David Kuehn, a cigar maker.

He was born in 1830 near Big Rock on the Lehigh Mountain south of Allentown. He grew up in poverty.

When cigar making was slow in Allentown, he went to Connecticut for a time to pursue his trade there, then returned to care for his aged parents.

Late in life, he married Sallie Ann Wieder. They had no children.

Life was a struggle for him, and this is what helped him feel so keenly for the crippled orphan children at The Good Shepherd Home.

His prosperity came when he bought eleven acres at Fourteenth and Chew streets, which he turned into a truck patch and afterward sold to a real estate company for $35,000.

He reinvested that money wisely in Allentown property. He acquired twenty-one houses.

Somewhere around 1912, when the Home was just four years old, Papa was on his way by train from Allentown to Reading when he met Dr. John A. Singmaster, president of the Lutheran Theological Seminary at Gettysburg. Singmaster was traveling to his old home in Macungie.

The good doctor had greatly helped Papa in the campaign to remove the debt from the Topton Orphans' Home and had a wonderful insight into

111

financial things concerning the Lord's work.

Singmaster asked, "Do you know David Kuehn of Allentown?"

Papa didn't.

Singmaster said, "Mr. Kuehn was a member of St. Paul's Lutheran Church, but for some reason became estranged. I can't handle him. But probably you can influence him."

As a result, Papa called on Kuehn about twice a year. Kuehn listened to Papa's story and asked many questions, but that's about all the encouragement he gave.

With the 1916 campaign for $100,000, Papa and a committee visited Kuehn. But the man said he could not do anything then, but after his death something would come and the Home would be satisfied.

He said he had implicit confidence in what the board would do.

David Kuehn died in April 1919 and his wife in June 1922, both listed as members of the Mennonite Church. With her death, their wealth went to Good Shepherd. It was about $100,000. At the time, it was one of the largest bequests ever to a Lutheran institution of mercy.

The Kuehn money was used to pay the bulk of the first phase of the building project—the $125,000 dormitory for sixty boys, dedicated in August 1923.

The board called the dormitory the Kuehn Memorial Building.

Ironically, Mr. Kuehn originally had the Gettysburg Seminary in his will, but changed it and substituted The Good Shepherd Home. Dr. Singmaster was big-hearted enough not to feel hurt, Papa said.

One footnote to that 1920 go-around with the Medical Society:

In 1954, the Lehigh County Medical Society honored The Good Shepherd Home with a Benjamin Rush Award—given for providing outstanding health and welfare services to the community. The society particularly cited Good Shepherd for offering those services to the physically handicapped without regard to race, creed or color. ❖

The Good Shepherd Home is laying the groundwork for still more difficult work.

Sweet Charity
July-August 1917

Papa Raker tried his best to tie The Good Shepherd Home with bits of history. This helped to advertise the cause.

He hailed the "firsts" or the "oldests" in almost everything that was connected to the Home.

The Home, of course, was the first of approximately fifty Lutheran institutions in America to take in crippled children and infants, able-bodied or disabled.

It was also the first Lutheran home to send its children to the public schools.

Aunt Mary Eisenhard, the first aged person admitted to the Home, just happened to be the first teacher in Lehigh County to use the blackboard—a fact Papa readily shared with *Sweet Charity* readers.

Today, we would also hail Aunt Mary as probably the first feminist in the old Evangelical Lutheran Ministerium of Pennsylvania, which covered the eastern third of the state. When the learned clergy of her day told her not to start a Women's Missionary Society in the Allentown Conference, she ignored them and went ahead and did it anyway.

Papa had some choice comments for *Sweet Charity* readers in those early years about some wealthy institutions that were caring for orphans. Their narrow ways showed just why Good Shepherd had to be first in some of the things it was doing.

The real object of an institution, Papa said, is not to erect great buildings or secure large endowments, "but to do a great service for mankind." Love and mercy are essential. The buildings and endowment are simply tools to carry out that love and mercy. Connie and Dale still echo those words.

"Another essential thing for an institution to succeed in the highest sense with respect to the children is to have the love, sympathy and cooperation of the community and the public," Papa said.

This cannot be secured when there is no need and when the public can't help or take an active part in its support and management.

He pointed *Sweet Charity* readers to the five leading orphanages of the day as far as financial resources were concerned. And he cited some things that wouldn't hit home in the courts or in the American sense of fair play for another forty years.

But, after all, Papa was something of an Old Testament prophet. Here, prophet Raker was speaking in 1924:

GIRARD COLLEGE—Founded by Stephen Girard, located in the center of Philadelphia on forty-five acres, surrounded by a huge stone wall ten feet high. It opened in 1848.

According to Girard's will, the home took poor white male orphans between six and ten years. They could remain until at least fourteen but not beyond eighteen. The courts had said an orphan means fatherless.

"When Girard College celebrates its centennial in 1948, it has been predicted the endowment will reach one hundred million," Papa said.

"Stephen Girard had only one eye, but he could see further than most people with two. His will, the expression of his desire to help the poor orphan boy, is as far in advance of his day and generation as it is lacking in our day.

"Millions and stone walls will not be permitted to separate the future orphan boy from the best that can be secured for him in the pliant years of his life.

114

"Girard College has done a great work and will continue to do a still greater work.

"If the ten-foot-high stone wall is not removed by the centennial year 1948, it will be removed by the time the second centennial takes place."

That stone wall is still there in 1988 and an official at Girard claims it will be there for the 200th anniversary. But a militant, abrasive and undaunted black attorney in Philadelphia named Cecil Moore led picketers around that stone wall and carried a legal suit all the way to the U.S. Supreme Court until the walls of racial segregation tumbled down at that institution in 1968.

The so-called functional orphan, where a parent was not being a parent, was admitted in 1977 and girls were accepted starting in 1984. Girls comprise about a fifth of the 500 resident students.

Yes, the endowment is well over $100 million.

To anyone reading these words in 2048, you'll know if prophet Raker's prediction about the stone wall itself has been fulfilled.

HERSHEY INDUSTRIAL SCHOOL—Founded by chocolate manufacturer Milton S. Hershey about a mile south of Hershey, Pennsylvania. In 1909, Hershey and his wife gave title to 486 acres for the orphanage. Hershey's estate, estimated at over sixty million, is to be given to the home.

Hershey School received poor white healthy orphan boys between four and eight. They were indentured to age eighteen.

Papa observed, "If Mr. Hershey made any mistakes with respect to his will, he has the advantage over Stephen Girard because he is still living and can change them."

The change, of course, was not to be during Hershey's lifetime. Like Girard College, Hershey admitted the first black in 1968.

And in 1977, the school successfully petitioned the court to redefine orphans as children not receiving adequate care from their natural parents.

CARSON COLLEGE—Robert N. Carson left an estate of $3.5 million for this home. Only full orphan white girls—that is, girls who have lost both father and mother—between ages six and ten were accepted.

"It is a question whether that home can find such girls to comply with the demands of the will," Papa observed. "It plainly shows Carson did not know the great needs of the day."

Full orphan girls between six and ten are seldom in need of a home, Papa said. In his almost twenty-five years as superintendent at Topton and now Good Shepherd, involving thousands of applications, he had not had a half dozen for healthy full orphan girls between six and ten.

Now called Carson Valley School at Flourtown, Pennsylvania, it survived through the 1950s under its original terms, then had the courts broaden its mandate. It now handles neglected and dependent children, some temporarily for evaluation, some residential with a school on the grounds. Some ninety-five percent of the youngsters are blacks.

MOOSEHEART—This home is at Mooseheart, Illinois, thirty miles west of Chicago, on 1,023 acres of the best land in the world. It was sustained by $2 annual dues from the Loyal Order of Moose, roughly $1 million in 1924.

Membership in the Moose rose dramatically with the start of Mooseheart. One of its leading spirits was U.S. Labor Secretary James J. Davis.

The home took babies as well as older children whose parents died in good standing in the organization.

One factor Papa omitted to mention was that the Moose was limited to whites. After 1973, the Moose removed Caucasian from its membership limitations, and Virginia McGowan at the home reports Mooseheart has several blacks among its 300 youngsters.

The support is now $8 a year from Moose members for both Mooseheart and Moosehaven, facilities in Florida for the elderly.

Since its beginnings, the widow of a Moose member and her children could live at Mooseheart until the children finished high school. Now, the home also

116

takes the functional orphans—children of divorced parents, handicapped parents and such.

HASTINGS-ON-HUDSON—This orphanage of the Orphan Society of New York City came into existence in 1806. It was originally on Riverside Drive in Manhattan, then in 1902 moved up the Hudson.

"This is one that tries to adapt itself to the real needs of children," said Papa, who had seen all five. "They have the best cottage system to be found."

This home receives healthy orphans and half-orphans between three and ten.

Today, this is the Graham-Windham Services to Families and Children. It is a foster care agency for unwanted, neglected and abused children from metropolitan New York. It has 160 living on the campus, which also has its own school. The population is sixty-five percent black and thirty percent Hispanic.

In 1924, the St. John Street prophet concluded, "You will observe that the most needy, helpless, homeless orphan children, the crippled, the blind, the epileptic and the sickly, who cannot be placed in private families, are not even considered at any age by the five leading orphanages of the country.

"Not one of the crippled, blind, epileptic, sickly orphan or destitute children of The Good Shepherd Home could have been admitted by any of these five homes. It seems as if the millions and the really needy orphan child had no connections.

"This will not always be so.

"The need of the most helpless orphan children is slowly but surely being brought to the attention of the future philanthropist, and he will not, he cannot ignore them.

"Even the priest and the Levite will not continue to pass by on the other side."

* * *

Papa had a story for just about everything, including one about the first bequest that was bestowed upon Good Shepherd. It came from a member of his first congregation in Pen Argyl.

117

If ever there was a place where Papa loved the people and where he had strong reason to feel the people loved him, it was in that small community in eastern Pennsylvania at the foot of the Blue Mountain.

Papa got to Pen Argyl by accident.

While at seminary, he filled in for a classmate on May 20, 1891, who was to supply-preach for the mission, St. John's, at Pen Argyl. "We came, we saw, we conquered and were conquered," Papa recalled.

The congregation wanted him to supply that summer. Papa did and then once a month during his senior year at seminary. After graduation, he became the first regular pastor to St. John's. The mission soon became self-supporting. Papa stayed seven years.

One of Papa's first converts was John Winsborough, one of the pioneer slaters from England to America. He worked in the slate quarries of Pen Argyl for a number of years. Being a good worker and having good business sense, he amassed a considerable fortune through investments in real estate.

He married rather late in life to a widow who subsequently died before he did. They had no children.

Winsborough was rough natured, but tender-hearted. "He had fallen into the drinking habit, and it was here where his faithful wife and the grace of God helped to make a man of him," Papa said.

Winsborough was almost sixty when he was confirmed. Conversion turned him into a total abstainer from intoxicating liquors. Papa, the prohibitionist, was delighted.

Winsborough never missed a service, even when an occasional German sermon was preached.

When Papa asked why he attended the service when he did not understand it, Winsborough replied, "The service was all in English, except the sermon, and thus I could be greatly benefited. Besides, I started late in life and did not want to miss a service."

The Winsboroughs became like mother and father to Papa.

With the start of The Good Shepherd Home, Winsborough revised his will to include it along with other money for his church and Lutheran foreign missions.

The man died in early 1910. His provision for Good Shepherd amounted to about $4,000. That was at a time the Home had an annual income of around $10,000.

Six others had already included the Home in their wills, some drawn up before Winsborough. He happened to be the first among that group to die.

The 1912 Christmas issue of *Sweet Charity* noted the first bequest from someone outside the Lutheran Church. This was $500 from the estate of Mary Ann Spinner of Spinnerstown, a village in Bucks County about ten miles south of Allentown. She was a member of the Reformed Church.

Papa soon adopted a ritual at the Anniversary Day program of having the names read of those who had provided bequests in the prior year and the amount their wills had bestowed upon the Home. They would be listed in the subsequent issue of *Sweet Charity*. It was a practice that was carried on for years.

Good Shepherd also had among its firsts the blind widow of the first Union soldier to fall in the battle of Gettysburg.

Diana Sandoe, a Methodist, entered the Home July 14, 1914, and died there December 17, 1915. She was buried in Gettysburg. She had been blind for twenty-five years.

Her husband George was the first man killed on the battlefield of Gettysburg, a member of the Twenty-first Pennsylvania Volunteer Cavalry. Such note was taken of this fact that two monuments were erected near the spot where he fell.

Sandoe, with another Union cavalryman, was on a scouting tour down the Baltimore Road just outside Gettysburg. Sandoe dismounted while his comrade continued down the road. He encountered a Confederate cavalryman, fired at him and received a fatal bullet in exchange. The inscription on his unit's monument, located near Spangler's Spring, reads: "Near this spot on June 26, 1863, fell Private George W. Sandoe, an advance scout of a company of

119

volunteer cavalry, afterwards Company B, Twenty-five Pennsylvania Cavalry. The first Union soldier killed at Gettysburg.''

* * *

A swindler by the name of John Eberoth of Hellertown joined the ranks of Good Shepherd firsts in 1914—the first person caught collecting money fraudulently in the Home's name.

Almost from the Home's founding, Papa had warned contributors to send checks, not cash, when they mailed in gifts.

The cash didn't always reach its destination, and he claimed there was some elbowing among Post Office people to get the route that included Good Shepherd.

But here with Eberoth was open thievery.

As *The Morning Call* reported in June 1914, Eberoth had been operating in quite a number of towns in this section, soliciting money for the Home.

When he came to a certain place in South Bethlehem some weeks earlier, suspicion was at once directed toward him. The South Bethlehem police chief arrested him, charging him with getting money under false pretenses.

A magistrate gave Eberoth three months in jail and a fine of $25. Papa had been one of those called to testify in the case.

Through the newspaper, Papa let it be known that ''no person is at present collecting money for the institution and nobody should be led into any of the snares of frauds.''

Sweet Charity did not share this case with its readers.

But Papa really waded in when Oscar Krasley, a Pentecostal minister from Allentown, worked the same racket several years later. Papa seemed absolutely gleeful in reporting to the board in early 1919: ''We finally succeeded in capturing Rev. Krasley who has been collecting funds for at least two years, without authority, for Good Shepherd and without ever giving the Home a cent.''

Papa had warned *Sweet Charity* readers in the

summer of 1918 in a segment simply labeled FRAUD:

"An unauthorized person is reported to have collected money in the name of The Good Shepherd Home for crippled children in Allentown. Reports have come from Schuylkill Haven, Orwigsburg, Robesonia, Womelsdorf, Myerstown, Birdsboro, Reading and Topton, etc.

"The party has a paper covered booklet called 'The Way of Salvation' with a picture of J.W. Krasley of Allentown. We called to see Mr. Krasley on North Tenth Street. Mr. Krasley denies any knowledge of such false representations. He admits he is the author of the booklet which contains his picture."

Papa concluded: "Help The Good Shepherd Home arrest this religious fraud who has collected a great deal of money of which the Home never received a cent."

Papa didn't tell *Sweet Charity* readers at the time that Krasley's booklet called Lutheran preachers blind leaders of the blind. But that attack may have accounted in part for Papa's rejoicing over Krasley's being caught.

Krasley's downfall was in collecting thirty cents from a woman in Fountain Hill and putting the money in his pocket without making a record of the name and amount. The woman phoned the Home. When Papa heard the woman had received Krasley's booklet, he knew who the culprit was and phoned authorities.

Krasley spent two nights in jail before having to face a dozen witnesses who testified they gave him money for Good Shepherd. Justice of the Peace W.H. Stahlnecker said he could have secured two dozen more to testify.

Krasley pleaded guilty "to soliciting funds throughout the country for The Good Shepherd Home for which he had no authority." Stahlnecker extracted from the defendant a promise never to sell his booklet again nor collect funds for Good Shepherd.

The JP sentenced him to nine months in jail and fined him $200, then suspended sentence "on condition he stop peddling, preaching and collecting and secure honest labor to support himself and his family." Further, Krasley had to report to the squire once a month for two years.

* * *

On a more uplifting note, to The Good Shepherd Home Band went two titles of "oldest."

It had the oldest director in Pennsylvania in Joseph Smith who served the band until his death at age eighty-five and it posed on several occasions with Clover, the Methuselah of the horse world, owned by the Rev. Uriah Myers, pastor emeritus of St. Matthew's Lutheran Church of Catawissa, Pennsylvania. That's right, with the oldest horse in the world, whose celebrated presence was exhibited in Madison Square Garden in May 1922 and whose celebrated remains were given to the American Museum of Natural History in New York upon Clover's passing on April 26, 1924, at age fifty-three.

The band with Clover was pictured in *Sweet Charity*. The band with Clover was on postcards to publicize the Home.

Surely, Papa was the P.T. Barnum of the Lutheran Church.

The band was started in early 1915 with an optimistic announcement in *Sweet Charity* simply labeled: THE GOOD SHEPHERD HOME BAND.

Papa admitted the headline looked good, sounded good and some day would be a reality. Seventeen youngsters were ready to join. Smith, director of the famous Allentown Juvenile Band as well as a number of other bands, "examined our boys and says we have better material than he had when he started the Juvenile Band."

Sweet Charity provided a gift list of nineteen instruments needed of nine different varieties—from one bass drum with cymbals to five B-flat cornets.

But apparently nothing was done about the band for four years. Then in 1919, pictures of the band-in-the-making made the cover of three consecutive issues of *Sweet Charity*.

The formidable Joseph Smith was pictured in a studio shot with twenty-five boys from the Home in

122

their Sunday best finery who were called the "raw recruits for The Good Shepherd Home Band." It was a goodly number considering the Home had a total of sixty-five children of all ages at the time.

The cutlines said Smith has been engaged to teach them and predicted they will be able to play for the eleventh Anniversary Day that August 14. Four boys weren't on the picture because they were in the Orthopedic Hospital in Philadelphia.

The lead story of the issue announced that a society for the band was organized to provide it with instruments, music, teacher and uniforms. It was headed by Robert A. Wagner, superintendent of Grace Lutheran Sunday School in Allentown, with Mama Raker as secretary and George Feehrer as treasurer. Feehrer was superintendent of Grace Lutheran Sunday School in Bethlehem.

The first practice was on May 23.

The band society punned that the musically inclined should get on the band wagon with contributions to help outfit the unit. Instruments alone were costing $550.

"Stop, look and listen," *Sweet Charity* urged. "When you hear or imagine you hear sweet sounds or strange discords, just say to yourself and your friends: 'It is The Good Shepherd Home Band getting ready for the eleventh Anniversary Day and nothing more.' "

The subsequent issue of *Sweet Charity* showed the band from long distance—across the waters of the Little Lehigh at the boys' summer campsite, rehearsing at streambank.

That was the first summer the boys were to have a camp along the Little Lehigh. George Tamke, a Mt. Airy Theological student and later a member of the Home's Advisory Board, was their supervisor.

Their daily fare included an afternoon "musical feast" with Director Smith to prepare for Anniversary Day.

The Pregnant Thoughts section of that issue of *Sweet Charity* offered some comments on the band:

—The newly organized band at The Good Shepherd Home will be one of the great attractions of

Anniversary Day.

—The band is such an attraction that people stop on the streets to listen to our boys.

—Some call The Good Shepherd Home Band the crippled band. We do not like that name.

Finally, in the July-August issue that included the Anniversary Day report, the band is shown with "leader, caretaker and superintendent" in what appear to be sailor hats, white shirts and wide ties—if not uniforms, certainly an outfit that could pass for uniforms.

The Anniversary Day story said the band of crippled boys "certainly was the chief attraction of the day."

The band members took their first extended trip in 1921—to Tamaqua, Stone Valley and Sacramento in the hard coal regions. They got lost in the darkness on the way and had to light a copy of *Sweet Charity* as a torch while one boy climbed the road sign to read what it said. Papa, of course, managed to have a camera available to record the event and use the photograph on the cover of the next issue.

Part of the entourage traveled in a bus of the Allentown moving firm of D. Jacoby and Sons, which had a motto spread across the side that read: "The World Moves, So Do We."

The band played at Dinkey Memorial Church in Ashfield, a church erected by Eurana Schwab, the wife of Bethlehem Steel magnate Charles Schwab . . . at the public square at high noon in Tamaqua . . . at Stone Valley in Northumberland County at an all-day program.

The offerings received totaled about $235. In addition, several hundred subscriptions were secured for *Sweet Charity*.

The account of the trip in *Sweet Charity*, probably written by Clarence Nissley, "our Horace Greeley," ended by saying this was a "never-to-be-forgotten trip in which the Home was shown marked kindness."

That fall, the children of the Home were taken in vans and cars to visit the Gen. Harry Clay Trexler deer and buffalo park in the hilly upper reaches of Lehigh County, a location that became a county park thanks to the general's will.

As part of the trip, the Home band played for the buffalo. In response, "the buffaloes made strange maneuverings," *Sweet Charity* reported.

The Good Shepherd Home Band and Clover, the horse, met and posed together for the first time during the band's second annual trip through the coal regions in the summer of 1922.

Home boy Clarence Nissley, who wrote the account of the trip for *Sweet Charity*, seemed matter-of-fact about Clover, saying only that the band and Clover met and posed for pictures for *Sweet Charity* and postal cards. "Clover is fifty-one years old," Nissley summarized.

After all, what can you say about an old horse once you've said it's old?

But Nissley had other observations about the trip:

. . . Traffic would be halted while the band played in town squares or on the steps of courthouses . . .

. . . At Mahanoy City, the band was treated to dinner by a merchant named Metzger. Afterward, the band gave a short concert at his house.

"We wondered why he was so willing to give the whole band such a splendid dinner himself, and we found out he had a crippled child himself. We are told that many of the best supporters of The Good Shepherd Home are those who have crippled children themselves . . ."

. . . Farmer Alex Billmeyer, eighty-one, of Washingtonville invited the band into his house and played a song on the fiddle from his boyhood days, "Washington's Grand March." Billmeyer "plays with the speed and fire of a young man . . ."

. . . The boys of the band seemed "enraptured by the pretty girls" around Numidia . . .

. . . The band visited Frank E. DeLong, the inventor of the hook and eye . . .

. . . Eva Pauley found and read favorite passages from the Gospels of Luke and John to members of the audience.

"Miss Pauley also gave a demonstration of how a blind person can operate any standard typewriter. The

Royal Typewriter Co. of Allentown supplied the Home with a new typewriter and case for the trip."

. . . The trip covered 250 miles, produced $972 in offerings against $135 in expenses and brought 329 subscriptions to *Sweet Charity*. "We were all delighted with the opportunity to see what we saw."

The band took a second trip that summer—through the heartland of the Pennsylvania Dutch country. And it was a history trip for the youngsters as much as a chance to perform.

They visited Conrad Weiser's grave, Mama's most famous ancestor; orphan homes at Topton, Middletown, Hershey and Womelsdorf; the Cornwall iron mines where they were taken 800 feet down into a sloped mine, and the state capitol.

Along the way they received a donation of $1,800 from Philip A. Urich of Millersville, Lancaster County, for band instruments. To show their thanks, they serenaded Urich and his wife at their home.

Nearly 400 miles. Counting the money for the band instruments, income of $3,944 against expenses of $160.

Girls finally made it into the band itself in 1923. And as Roberta (Raker) Hudders recalls, the girls were sitting inside the band bus at the windows while the boys were seated on chairs outside for the traditional picture with Clover.

Dr. Uriah Myers, Clover's owner, was writing a book about the horse, including in it a short sketch of Good Shepherd.

Papa suggested that Dr. Myers split the profits.

There was a trip through the coal regions, over 500 miles, including a stop at Frackville, the birthplace of Harry Filer, the Home's Caruso. A large crowd went wild over him when he sang.

At Susquehanna University, where the band played to a crowded chapel, a professor introducing Papa Raker claimed honors for himself, because Mama was a former student of his at Myerstown.

Clarence Nissley reported offerings for the trip amounted to $3,197. The trips were now covering the Home's operating deficit.

Sweet Charity carried something of a postscript right under his detailed report:

"Even the street car conductors told us that it was lonesome at Sixth and St. John streets when our band was away on its trips through the coal regions."

There was a second trip that summer, through the Pennsylvania Dutch heartland like the previous year, part concert tour and part history lesson.

Eva Pauley, the blind girl, bumped her head on a low entranceway at the Ephrata Cloisters.

At Richland, the town's fire alarm was sounded to alert the populace to the concert. "In less than fifteen minutes, the whole town, factories and all, were ready for the concert," Nissley reported.

"This plan was so effective that our superintendent suggested other towns ring the fire alarm when we were ready to give concerts, but it seemed the people did not have the mutual understanding Richland had."

More than $3,000 in gifts, over 600 subscribers to *Sweet Charity,* over 500 miles traveled.

There was the coal regions trip in 1924 and then a series of short trips in various directions, netting $3,500. Clover's picture from 1922 ran for the last time in *Sweet Charity.* Readers were advised if they wanted to see Clover again, they should go to the American Museum of Natural History.

The band limped along for a number of years after that. But some of its members were through school and on their way out into life—the main goal that Good Shepherd had for them.

Papa put this footnote to Clarence Nissley's report of the 1924 trip:

"The children at The Good Shepherd Home will very likely forget many of the things that took place at the Home, but we feel confident that the band trips will not be forgotten." ❖

13: BEQUESTS LOST AND GAINED

The Lord has not always given us what we asked, but He generally gives us what we need for His helpless, homeless children.

Sweet Charity
January-February 1915

Papa said God knew what He was doing when He didn't grant him all he asked.

There were a lot of things that just didn't work out the way Papa originally wanted. Some were outright disappointments. Some turned into huge blessings. All were usually highly public because Papa was one to lay his dreams and expectations out onto the pages of *Sweet Charity*.

Take two financial examples—the estates of Preston Lynn, the John Wanamaker store executive who died in 1926, and Henry Trexler, an Allentown hotel proprietor who died in 1904 while Papa and Mama were still running the Topton Orphanage.

Sweet Charity early on had warned there were people who said they planned to revise their wills to include Good Shepherd, only to die before they did so.

Don't procrastinate, Papa openly advised.

Preston Lynn was a local boy who made good in the big city and in the heart of a lot of local youngsters amid that success. He became manager of the John

Wanamaker store in New York City in 1902 and held that post until his death in 1925 in his Park Avenue home.

His funeral in Manhattan attracted New York Governor Al Smith and former New York Mayor John Hylan. More than a hundred Wanamaker people and others accompanied the body on a special train to Allentown for a second service in Zion Reformed where the honorary pallbearers included Gen. Harry Clay Trexler.

Hundreds of children from Jefferson School were let out of class to line the route from the church to Fairview Cemetery. And at the conclusion of the rites at the Lynn mausoleum, each youngster paraded forward to put a flower on the coffin.

This was the same cemetery where many Good Shepherd infants and elderly were laid to rest in donated graves.

Lynn came from Danielsville, a country village at the base of the Blue Mountain, the youngest of six children in a poor family. He had only six years of schooling. Yet, as Papa said, "Nature with the Christian graces endowed him with love, kindness, tenderness and insight that is not vouchsafed to all."

As a youngster, he worked as a clerk in stores in the Lehigh River village of Treichlers, Summit Hill and Allentown. He was a born businessman.

In 1891, he joined Wanamakers in Philadelphia at $10 a week. He soon came into the good graces of founder John Wanamaker and his son Rodman. He was transferred to New York in 1895.

Lynn was credited with putting Al Smith into office as governor of New York for the first time. He promoted the idea of the "brown derby" for Smith as a sign of an old-fashioned New York boy and used "East Side, West Side" as a campaign song in the final days of the election. He pushed Smith for president in 1920 and 1924.

He was also an organizer and treasurer of the Millrose Games, a Wanamaker-sponsored track and field meet held in the old Madison Square Garden.

Somehow, he considered Allentown his hometown.

In 1923, he arranged a relay run by 300 Allentown boys to carry a message from Mayor Malcolm Gross to New York Mayor Hylan. On another occasion, he was host to a large number of Allentown men at the Millrose Games.

A few years before Lynn died, Papa was invited to supply-preach at St. Paul's Lutheran Church at Indianland where Lynn's mother lived and belonged. Afterward, a councilman asked Papa to visit Mother Lynn since she was sick and there was no regular minister for the congregation. Papa went.

Sometime after the visit, Lynn sent contributions to Good Shepherd ranging from $100 to $500 and large stockings filled with presents for young and old alike at Christmas.

Once, Papa took Harry Filer, the Home's best singer, and Eva Pauley to sing for Lynn's mother when Lynn was present. That pleased the woman and her son immensely.

Papa visited Lynn in his New York office four days before he made his last will. Lynn asked a lot of questions about the Home. He pointed to a copy of *Sweet Charity* on his office table, "It was *Sweet Charity* that first drew me to The Good Shepherd Home."

Then, Lynn pointed his finger at Papa and said, "And what will become of The Good Shepherd Home when you die?"

Papa replied, "The Home has a host of friends far and wide. Organized efforts are made through centurion bands and ladies' auxiliaries pledged to increase support.

"We have faithful consecrated helpers who do more for the love of Christ in caring for the helpless ones than people will ordinarily do for the love of money.

"And we have trustees who are alert, efficient, staunch, faithful and true, working without remuneration. Where others made a fortune for themselves, the board made a fortune for The Good Shepherd Home."

Papa concluded, "God's work does not depend on one man. He buries the workman and carries on the work. When you and I die, the need for Christ-like help will continue."

Lynn dropped his hand, smiled and said, "I guess you are about right."

The Lynn will provided liberal bequests to relatives and friends. Then, it said, "All the rest, residue and remaining of my property, both real, mixed and personal, I give, devise and bequeath unto The Good Shepherd Home of Allentown, Pa."

As *Sweet Charity* proclaimed, "After personally observing and thoroughly investigating The Good Shepherd Home for over ten years, Mr. Lynn made the Home the one and only object of charity by giving his entire residuary estate to the Home.

"Just what the bequest will amount to is not definitely known at this time."

The way Papa had understood it from Lynn in that final meeting was that Good Shepherd was to receive Lynn's Briarcliff estate up the Hudson and some bonds. Sale of the three-acre estate alone would bring Good Shepherd perhaps as much as $100,000.

Papa initially reported to the board, "We have reason to believe this will be the largest bequest ever given to an American Lutheran institution of mercy."

But it turned out those liberal bequests to relatives and friends—which totaled more than $260,000— wiped out virtually all the cash in the estate. In addition, there were unpaid fees for the executors and their attorney totaling $55,000.

As Papa warned *Sweet Charity* readers at one point, "The Preston Lynn bequest will not turn out as we had expected. We are realizing that even in charitable work it is best not to count the eggs until they are laid and the chickens until they are hatched."

The Home was left with a choice that was really no choice:

—Dig in your own pocket and pay off the rest of the estate's bills. That would allow the Home to hang onto Briarcliff, hoping to sell it at a good price later to recoup those payouts and have some left over for the Home.

—Take $5,000 offered by the heirs and walk away

from it all. Let the heirs take their chances on what they will net from a forced sale now. And "now" had stretched out to late 1928.

The board reluctantly took the $5,000.

Papa spelled the whole thing out in the January-February 1929 issue of *Sweet Charity*. "The Home was mentioned as residuary legatee. Residuary means what is left, and, strictly speaking, there was nothing left."

* * *

The Henry Trexler estate was something in the shadows for decades.

Henry A. Trexler, an Allentown hotelman, and his wife, Annie, were tremendously fond of children, but had none of their own. They were members of Christ Reformed Church.

They built the Trexler House, later called the Sterling Hotel, in 1890 across the street from the Central Railroad terminal at the lower end of Allentown. Henry also ventured into real estate, so much so that he retired from the hotel business in 1901 to devote full time to his real estate holdings.

Henry Trexler died in 1905.

He left his life estate to his father and his widow. Upon their passing, the residuary estate (there's that term again) would go to the mayor of Allentown to be used immediately to found a Protestant orphans' home in the city.

Papa was at Topton at the time Trexler died. A member of that board speculated that if Trexler had been properly approached, the money would have gone to Topton.

Someone reminded Papa of the will shortly before the residuary provision took effect. Papa copied the document and consulted the Home's lawyer, Edwin Kline, suggesting the money go for a Trexler memorial at Good Shepherd, should the mayor be willing. Kline agreed.

In 1914, Papa visited Mayor Charles Rinn who knew nothing about the responsibilities being bestowed upon him under the Trexler will.

Papa told the mayor the $70,000 in the trust fund wouldn't provide enough income to buy property, erect a building and endow it—the necessities for starting an orphanage. This seems now a rather strange argument coming from a man who started Good Shepherd with fifty cents.

Papa suggested to Rinn that the money go to Good Shepherd for a building in memory of Henry Trexler. And he reported afterward that the mayor said he would try to do that.

What Rinn actually did was tell the court he didn't want the responsibility of administering the trust. The court named a Henry Trexler board of trustees.

Those trustees consulted experts and concluded what Papa had long ago told the mayor—there was not enough money there to start an orphanage. This whole business dragged out over nearly twenty years. The trustees asked to be dissolved.

The upshot was that, virtually as a 1933 New Year's Day present, Judge Claude T. Reno issued a decree awarding what was then announced as $106,000 from the Henry Trexler trust to The Good Shepherd Home.

Reno said Good Shepherd was deemed the best institution to carry out the charitable intentions of Henry Trexler.

This was the first major court victory for young Attorney William Hudders, Papa Raker's son-in-law, Roberta Raker's husband. He would represent the home in legal matters for the next several decades.

"The Good Shepherd Home is a most worthy institution," the judge observed. "Its superintendent is a spiritual man of the highest attainments, and his institution is filling a great need and winning a notable place in the affections of the community.

"Indeed, one suspects that had The Good Shepherd Home been in existence when Henry Trexler wrote his will, he would have designated it as the almoner for his generosity."

What a delightful, rarely used term is "almoner"— one who dispenses charity.

Sweet Charity concluded, "The Good Shepherd Home feels grateful and thankful, but also realizes the additional responsibility to Almighty God."

It was the second largest estate the home had ever received, $86,000 in securities and $20,000 in real estate.

Ah, Good Shepherd was just rolling in wealth, right in the heart of the Depression. Those who had gossiped that line almost since the Home's founding now had something definite to point to.

The fact was that getting the Henry Trexler trust was more than "additional responsibility to God." It was a headache.

The real estate was vacant lots, which meant no income as against expenses for taxes and sometimes city utilities. The securities were mortgages on properties where payments were delinquent or properties themselves for rent that needed costly repairs.

Papa used a whole page of *Sweet Charity* in 1934 to show what a year's presence of the Henry Trexler trust had meant to Good Shepherd.

It showed a net income of $490.28.

* * *

Now, set these two "failures" against the dozens and dozens of bequests that have come to Good Shepherd, many of them smaller, that have helped enable this institution to survive and then grow.

Papa constantly preached that the Home had to make new friends because some of the old ones were dying off.

In May 1928, the twentieth anniversary year of the Home, Papa told the board, "The bequests for the Home are increasing. This is very encouraging. If it were not for this source of income, we would not be in the position we are, and most of our charitable institutions would be greatly handicapped.

"Most donors had some personal touch with the Home.

"Four years ago, I was in Lancaster and Lebanon counties for two days and felt somewhat discouraged because I apparently accomplished very little at the time.

134

"While in Lebanon, I asked Edward E. Miller, one of our members of the advisory board, for some additional names of prospective friends of the Home. Among others, he gave me the name of Mr. J.K. Laudermilch and accompanied me to see him. Laudermilch promised to do something for the Home.

"At the beginning of this month, the Home received a check for $2,000."

An unexpected gift like this, along with the known bequests, was helping the Home to meet its bills in major expansion projects.

As this is being written at the start of 1988, The Good Shepherd Home has just benefited by more than $900,000 in the distribution of the largesse of the late Harrison W. and Myrtie M. Prosser, a Lutheran couple who lived modestly in an apartment over the drugstore they began in 1918 in Hellertown. Even as an adult, Harrison Prosser continued to deliver newspapers, something he liked to talk about.

The Prossers amassed a multi-million-dollar fortune by buying stock in SmithKline, the drug people, when it was just beginning. In 1968, they established an irrevocable religious and charitable trust with an initial gift of 32,000 shares of SmithKline, then valued at $1,560,000.

For the next twenty years, the trust distributed more than $12 million.

The year 1988 meant the final distribution, and there was $7.2 million to be given out. The largest single allocation was $1,441,600 to the Lutheran Church in America.

Good Shepherd and the Lutheran Home at Topton shared the second spot, each receiving $901,000. Dale Sandstrom accepted on behalf of Good Shepherd at a luncheon following a service of Thanksgiving and Communion in Christ Lutheran Church in Hellertown, the home church of the Prossers.

There were gifts of $720,000 each to Muhlenberg College in Allentown and Muhlenberg Hospital Center in Bethlehem as well as lesser six-figure amounts to a host of other Lutheran and community institutions.

Harrison Prosser died in 1978 and his wife in 1982.

A niece called them "kind and sharing people, whose stewardship carried on to so many people."

Connie Raker had gone to the Prossers years ago, back before that irrevocable trust. "I heard what they had done for Muhlenberg, and I asked them: how about doing that for us?" Connie explained.

"If it had been up to Myrtie, she would have given us the whole kit and caboodle. She was all for Good Shepherd.

"You see, they had this big block of stock, and they gave it to Muhlenberg to hold for a number of years and use the earnings from it."

Connie visited the Prossers many times. The result was a prominent place for Good Shepherd in that final distribution.

* * *

One impending bequest that could be in the millions has spread across the tenure of all three administrators of Good Shepherd. And the full impact of it probably won't be felt until long after the Rev. Dale Sandstrom has moved on.

Perhaps someone reading these words in the year 2025 will know for certain.

There's a charitable time bomb sitting in Lancaster County that's set to go off sometime into the next century, and Good Shepherd stands to benefit handsomely from it.

This is the estate of Benjamin Franklin Herr, better known as B. Frank Herr.

He died on December 23, 1933. But the first mention of him in Good Shepherd records doesn't appear until November 1946. And in that, Connie Raker was correct in foreseeing that Good Shepherd would not receive any income from the Herr estate for forty years and even longer before the Home gets its share of the distribution of principal.

Connie Raker learned of Herr when he presented the cause of Good Shepherd at St. John's Lutheran Church in Columbia, Lancaster County, in that fall of 1946. It was then the church of the Rev. Frank Adler, a classmate of Connie's from seminary.

Herr was born in 1859 in Columbia. He started his sales career with the Columbia Grocery Co., but left town in his late twenties to seek his fortunes in Kansas where he married at age fifty and continued to reside until his wife's death in 1924.

Somehow, he had made a fortune in oil and lumber in Louisiana in the meantime.

Details are scarce even in this eightieth anniversary year about Herr. Nor does there seem to be any information on just how Herr encountered The Good Shepherd Home. It had to be during Papa's years.

In any case, after the death of Herr's wife, Delia, this prosperous businessman returned east to Harrisburg where his mother, a brother and two sisters were living.

His mother had been a founder of St. John's in Columbia and had selected the name, St. John's, for the congregation. She and the other family members were instrumental in having Herr direct some of his wealth to St. John's.

At that time, St. John's was considering remodeling its existing church. Instead, it built a new one.

Upon her death on New Year's Day 1928, Frank's mother was eulogized as "a vital factor in the erection of the new church." The Herr Memorial Chimes were dedicated later that year, a gift from Frank to the church.

The irony is that Frank Herr didn't visit the new St. John's to which he had contributed so much. He was frequently abroad in the years before his death in 1933.

Herr left approximately $750,000 in trust—a massive sum in Depression times.

Income was split fourteen ways—to thirteen relatives and friends for life and the fourteenth share to St. John's. Some of those thirteen were young people. None of the individuals was to get more than $6,000 a year. If there was an amount beyond that, it would go to St. John's.

As each of the thirteen died, the income was to be divided equally among the rest.

Once all the individuals have died, then the income

is to be split 50 percent to St. John's, 25 percent to the Columbia Hospital and 25 percent to The Good Shepherd Home—for twenty-one years.

After that, the principal is to be distributed to those three institutions in the same manner.

Here in Good Shepherd's eightieth year, there are eight individual heirs remaining, ranging in age from their early seventies to their late eighties. And the latest statement from Commonwealth National Bank of Harrisburg puts the principal of the estate at $4,750,000.

There are apparently no records to show how the cause of the crippled orphans reached and touched Frank Herr.

But *Sweet Charity* of September-October 1924 leaves us a haunting note published about the time he was moving back east: "Millions will come to The Good Shepherd Home as soon as the Home needs it."

❖

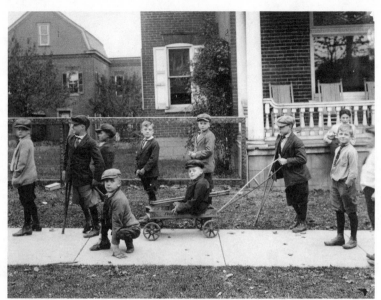

On the way to public school, 1917: Clarence Putt, Harry Filer, Norman Milander, Bill Remaley, Harold Romig, Clarence Nissley, John Yost, Bill Pitten and Eddie Shander. The little boy leaning against the fence is unknown.

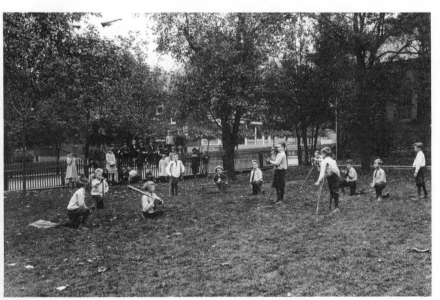

Batter up, 1917!

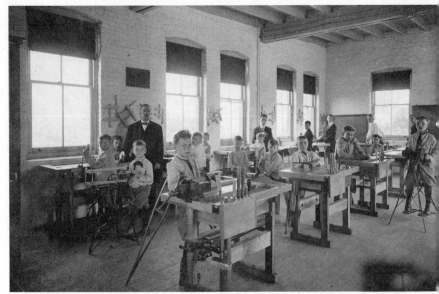

Vocational training at Good Shepherd, 1918.

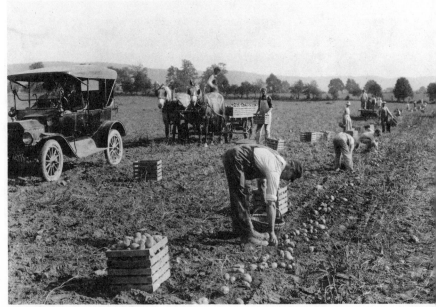

The Good Shepherd farm, 1918.

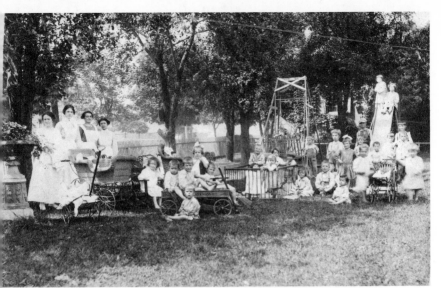

On the corner of The Good Shepherd Home lawn, 1919.

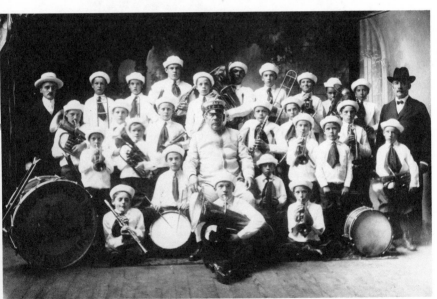

The Good Shepherd Boys Band led by Joseph Smith, 1919. Standing in front of Papa Raker, at the right, is young Connie Raker.

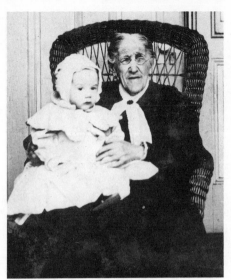

*"Aunt Mary" Eisenhard holds
Frank May, the first infant received
into The Good Shepherd Home,
1908.*

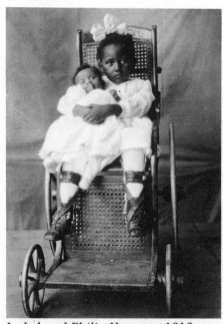

*Isabel and Philip Younger, 1919.
Despite criticism from some, Papa
Raker would tolerate no prejudices
at Good Shepherd.*

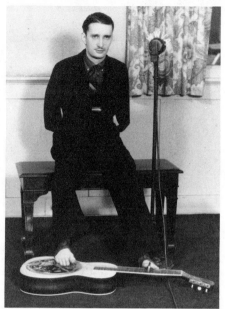

Armless Ray Myers grew up to be a successful musician and singer.

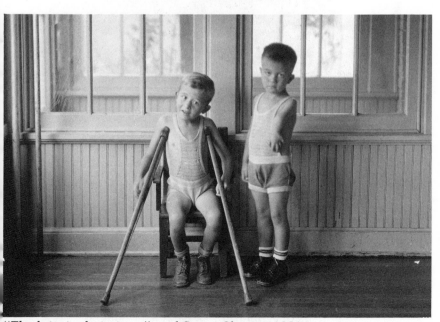

"The latest admissions," said Sweet Charity, 1931.

143

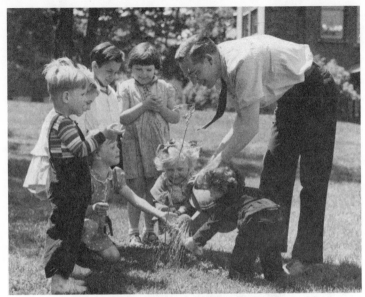

Connie Raker helps the little ones to plant a tree, 1945.

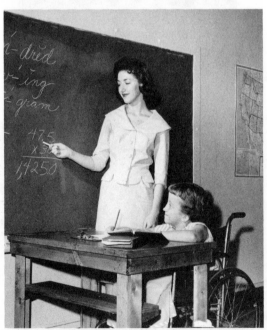

Education has always been a major priority at Good Shepherd. Teacher Sharon Kern and Maxine Mohn, 1960. Maxine became a teacher's aide in the 1980's.

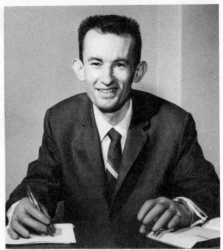

Dino Katsiaras lost both hands from a grenade explosion during the Communist uprising in Greece in the late 1940's. He spoke no English when he came to Good Shepherd, but went on to graduate from Muhlenberg College in 1963.

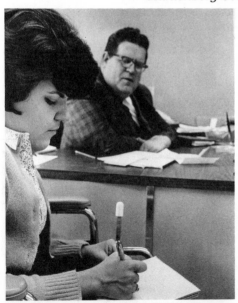

Raised at Good Shepherd, Carl Odhner went on to become a teacher and to be the founding director of Good Shepherd Vocational Services. Carl and Kathy Vastyshak, 1965.

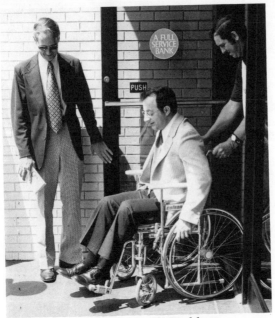

Allentown's Mayor Joseph Daddona experienced wheelchair barriers during "Roll on the Mall," 1973. Rehabilitation Hospital director Ray E. Crissey, left, lent a hand.

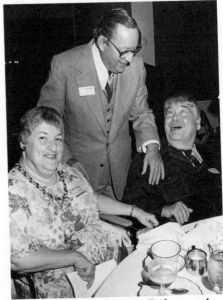

Delores Shook, Connie Raker and Eric Andrews, 1980.

There is some connection
between heaven and The
Good Shepherd Home.

Sweet Charity
September-October 1940

There seems to be no end to the stories that come
out of the early years of Good Shepherd. *Sweet
Charity* is filled with them. So are Papa Raker's
reports to the board. And, yet, there has to be a
moving on.

Connie Raker and Dale Sandstrom both deserve
considerable attention for their years as administrator.
After all, Connie headed the Home longer than Papa.
And in what so far has been a relatively few years,
Dale has presided over a virtual explosion of Good
Shepherd in size and scope.

Please permit, though, one last skip through those
earlier times—like the last sad walk through a house
that had served so well, to make sure the moving
people took everything.

The Rev. Herman Ernst Christman Wahrmann
arrived at Good Shepherd with wife and children to
accept a call as "administrative secretary" on Dec. 3,
1920, the day after his fifty-first birthday.

He remained active until almost the end of his life on
Oct. 8, 1968, at age ninety-eight. And though he never
served on the Good Shepherd board, he lived long
enough to see his son, the Rev. M. Luther Wahrmann,
join the board in 1959.

The elder Wahrmann was still going strong in the 1950s when Connie Raker told a friend, "Here I'm thinking about a pension plan for retired employees and I've got a man on the payroll who's in his eighties."

Rev. Wahrmann was five when his parents immigrated to America in 1873 from Germany. He grew up in New England. He worked as a weaver until he was twenty and continued to support himself through Wagner College. He was a graduate of Lutheran Seminary of Philadelphia, Class of 1897.

His pastoral ministry was all in the Danville Conference of the Ministerium of Pennsylvania—Lykens, Turbotville, Numidia, Lock Haven and Lykens again.

In 1912, he organized the Danville Conference Centurion Band, a group of one hundred individuals, Sunday schools and other groups who supported the purchase, renovation and expansion of an infants' cottage for Good Shepherd. They were to give five dollars a year for as long as they could for this work.

As chairman, Wahrmann had to visit the Home at least once a year and report back to the conference. It was through this work that the Home's advisory board recommended him and the trustees unanimously chose him as Good Shepherd's administrative secretary.

To provide for its new worker, the Home bought an eight-room house at 730 St. John Street for the Wahrmann family, cleaned it and put a ton of chestnut coal and forty-five bushels of potatoes (seconds) in the cellar. "We all tried to make his reception as pleasant as we possibly could," Papa said.

The first work to greet him was about 3,000 envelopes containing contributions, all tied in neat packages of about a hundred—response to the Thanksgiving-Christmas appeal.

Within a month, Papa would report to the board: "He is on the job and we are all pleased with the way he takes hold of the work. All is peace and harmony. He came at harvest time and is doing all that could be expected."

Wahrmann obviously was extra special. He smoked cigars, and Papa's stand against smoking had long been established.

A generation later, Connie Raker would be echoing Papa's praise of Wahrmann to the board: "Unless you are closely connected with the daily life of The Good Shepherd Home, you do not realize what a wonderful asset he is.

"Through the years, he has built up an efficient office organization. In addition to all the other functions, he has also cared for the investments of the Home under the finance committee."

Wahrmann was ensconced in office about two months when Papa walked in. Wahrmann said, "I'm not satisfied with the way the work is being done."

Papa looked at him, "What's the matter? Don't you like your job?"

Wahrmann: "The job is all right, but the manner of doing things here is antiquated and needs a thorough overhauling."

Papa: "Well, what do you want?"

Wahrmann said that what he had in mind was an addressograph that would cost $1,600.

Papa: "Map out your plans and present them to the board at the next meeting."

Wahrmann's part-time predecessor, the Rev. Jeremiah H. Ritter, kept the list of contributors in small books, arranged according to certain cities or localities. To find a contributor, Wahrmann first had to know where the individual lived and then locate the name in the appropriate small book. It was chaos.

He quickly went to an alphabetized card list.

"At this time, there were about 10,000 names on the mailing list," Wahrmann recalled. "When it was time to get out an issue of *Sweet Charity*, all had to be written by hand.

"Everyone around the place who could write legibly and Mrs. Raker was put to work. After about two weeks of moaning and groaning, the work was finally accomplished."

Besides being slow, the Ritter system was riddled with duplications. They showed up in going to an

149

alphabetized list.

Wahrmann called June 13, 1921, his lucky day. That was the day the addressograph arrived.

The next issue of *Sweet Charity* was addressed in less than two days.

When Good Shepherd built its rehabilitation hospital in 1964, it was Wahrmann at age ninety-four who was given the honor of turning the first shovelful of dirt.

*   *   *

Good Shepherd took the odds and ends of humanity under a variety of circumstances.

Sometimes, it accepted youngsters on a temporary basis because the father was working and the mother was in the hospital. This would go as planned—unless the mother died, which happened sometimes.

On occasion, it was a teen-age unmarried mother with her child—the babe cared for in the infants cottage while the mother worked for the Home. The same kind of thing would be done for impoverished widows with young children.

Just a smattering of the cases from Papa's reports to the board gives some idea of just how extensive was the mercy of Good Shepherd:

"Elizabeth Greenwood, wife of Dennis Ahner, one of the first orphans admitted to the Topton Home, died September 1, 1919, at the Hamburg Sanitarium, aged thirty years. Three of her children, Luther, Ella and Eva, are at the Home and have been here for five years. We took these children to witness the burial of their mother.

"These children are not crippled. Their case is peculiar and exceptional. When the father and mother were sick, they were received here because they were not orphans and could not be admitted in the regular orphanage.

"After the father was dead, application was made by the mother with our consent to have them admitted into the Topton Home. They were not received, and we kept them."

"Mary Briggs, one of our colored girls, entered the Home September 21 and left December 26, 1922. The mother, who had run away, came back and claimed the girl."

"William Remaley, one of our older boys, has been attending to the laundry since Mr. Henderson left. William's father paid ten dollars per month for his son at the Home. We recommend that the Home pay William ten dollars per month for his work." (October 13, 1924).

"Joseph Kirshen, crippled Hebrew boy six years of age from Allentown, entered December 2, 1924. Brother not being crippled entered Hebrew Home at Erie, Pennsylvania."

Joseph was taken by his mother June 20, 1925.

"Minnie Geist, born at Shamrock, Pennsylvania, March 4, 1913. Entered the Home September 15, 1916. The father, Franklin Geist, was killed on the railroad. The mother is dead. She comes from Rev. William F. Bond's congregation.

"She was refused admission into the Topton Home, because she could not walk. She wore braces for a number of years. The sister claims to be able to give her a good home and asks if she can get her by May or June (1925)."

Minnie left to live with her sister and aunt near Alburtis on July 4, 1925.

"We put an ad in the paper for a janitor. The first applicant was a colored gentleman named Clarence Lee, twenty-five. His recommendations were good. We engaged him at forty dollars a month and board." (May 12, 1924)

A subsequent report in spring 1925 showed that Lee and five children from the Home took catechetical instruction and were confirmed at Grace Lutheran.

"Verna Hoppes, the crippled girl, living six miles southeast of Tamaqua, was investigated March 18, 1925. The father and step-mother are living on a farm. The girl cannot be taken to school and for this reason application is made to The Good Shepherd Home.

"Like many farmers, the parents are in somewhat straitened circumstances and could not pay anything towards the child. They, however, promised to furnish the clothes."

"Kenneth Hartman from Litchfield, Ohio, entered October 2, 1925. This boy is doing very nicely. He lost one arm and one leg in an automobile and railroad accident in which his mother and sister were killed. This boy was strongly recommended by Daddy Allen, the first president of the International Society for Crippled Children."

"Clara Viola Shipe Pennypacker, one of our destitute girls, was placed in a family in Rev. Sandt's congregation, Catawissa, Pennsylvania, eleven years ago. This month, the mother, who is now married, inquired about the child for the first time.

"We informed her that her daughter was adopted in a splendid family where there were no children and had all the advantages of a Christian home and would some day inherit a small fortune. We did not tell her in our first letter where her daughter was and she has not inquired about her since." (December 14, 1925)

That seemed to confirm a decision the board made in May 1913: "It was moved that Clara Pennypacker of Trevorton, an inmate of our Home, not be given over to her mother, she being not a fit woman to have children."

Papa attended the convention of the United Lutheran Church at Richmond, Virginia, October 19 to 28, 1926. The copies of *Sweet Charity* that were distributed disappeared like magic.

The Rev. Dr. Robert W. Doty, a Lutheran pastor of Rochester, Pennsylvania, asked how Gerald Guinn was getting along. Gerald had been admitted some months earlier after a stint in jail.

Papa said the Home had done everything it possibly could for Gerald, but saw no special signs or indications it would succeed in making a saint out of him.

Dr. Doty replied, "Well, if you had, I would want to make application at The Good Shepherd Home myself."

"We went to New Holland where we presented the cause to the Lions Club. Over one hundred present, an excellent opportunity to present the cause.

"We investigated the case of the armless boy,

Raymond Myers, and took him with us on our continued trip. He entered the Home July 13, 1927."

"Miss Louise Leisenring brought Italian twins from Sacred Heart Hospital, Antonio and Anna Marie Josephine Petroccio, whose mother died at their birth. They were admitted to the baby cottage October 31, 1927, the father agreeing to pay five dollars per week."

"Two boys, Thomas Stank and John Lagouras, who were given into the care and keeping of Rev. Frederick Fasig, the Catholic missionary of South Allentown, are still at the Home. The priest has asked all their institutions, but none will accept the boys because they are crippled. He confesses that they had no institutions that would admit them." (November 12, 1928)

"Eric Andrews, born November 25, 1915, West Annapolis, Maryland, unable to walk, was brought here November 16, 1929, by Red Cross nurse. We permitted the boy to be brought here until the board meeting. In case he is not accepted, the Red Cross will take him away.

"He was brought to the Weidner School for Crippled Children in Philadelphia. They would not accept him because he is too helpless. They informed him of The Good Shepherd Home. Gen. Harry C. Trexler is interested in this case through a special friend of his in Philadelphia."

"Application: Mr. B.C. Stauffer of Coopersburg, age eighty-four, has $200 and his son will pay $500, clothe him, give him spending money and bury him when he dies. This is the man that gave all his money to his daughter to keep him for life and now she has nothing herself. Her husband is in jail." (March 11, 1930)

"Mr. Stauffer entered on April 2, 1930. The daughter where he stayed broke up housekeeping and is working at our baby cottage." (April 8, 1930)

Dr. George Gebert of Tamaqua, the board president, was authorized to go to Philadelphia and interview in the case of a blind and feeble-minded applicant asking admission into the old people's department. In this, Dr. Gebert had the power to act.

"The applicant arrived July 10, 1930. She is thirty-seven, a unique case and not suitable for our old people's home. This will have to be considered later.

"The person in question, Ella M. Mantz, was not admitted to the home for the blind because she was feeble-minded and was not admitted into the home for feeble-minded because she is blind."

"George Goldfus, twelve-year-old crippled boy of Lancaster, entered August 14, 1930."

"A baby from an unmarried Catholic girl from Easton was received December 31, 1937, until it can be placed for adoption."

* * *

Eric Andrews, William Remaley and George Goldfus would become fixtures at Good Shepherd. Verna Hoppes would grow up at the Home, get a degree from Cedar Crest, become employed, marry Home boy Clarence Putt and move on into a home of her own. And the Ahner children would blossom and go out in the world as well.

Eric Andrews had polio as an infant in 1916. In 1942, his right leg was amputated because of poor circulation, and he was not able to use his right arm.

But he turned out to be far from helpless in the fifty-three years he would live at Good Shepherd. When he first arrived, he asked: "Do they teach you to be an artist here?"

And the answer he got was "yes."

He developed into an artist and designer, operating a mail order firm for business cards, wedding announcements and personalized printing. He became the illustrator for *Sweet Charity*, the first to have a full color cover illustration in the magazine.

He was honored in 1979 as the "Voice of *Sweet Charity*."

Shortly before Papa Raker passed away in 1941, Eric thought of the idea of calling people daily to tell them about the work of Good Shepherd and, before hanging up, ask if they'd like to subscribe to *Sweet Charity*. It would be his way of thanking the Home for the care he had received.

Connie Raker was the one to grant Eric permission

to have his own phone installed.

"Every weekday since 1941, except when I was ill or away visiting relatives, I have devoted time to calling up people in the Lehigh Valley and surrounding areas. Each phone call is an adventure into the unexpected," Eric said near the end of his life.

"Most have heard about Good Shepherd, but are uncertain about the extent of our rehabilitation and residency programs. To anyone expressing an interest in Good Shepherd, I forward a sample of *Sweet Charity*. I estimate about fifty percent become subscribers."

Eric reached more than 400,000 people that way.

In the early 1940s, Eric also began to study art through a WPA recreation program and with sculptor William Roberts of Bethlehem. He became a member of the Lehigh Art Alliance, which met sometimes at Good Shepherd as an accommodation to him.

In 1946, he purchased a motorized wheelchair, a first at Good Shepherd, with money he raised by selling art and 10,000 religious bookmarks. It was a three-wheeler, gasoline powered, seventy-two miles a gallon, top speed of twenty-two miles an hour.

Eric's paintings and drawings were exhibited at many Allentown locations and in shows in New York City, New Orleans, Ohio and New Jersey.

In 1978, he produced a calendar featuring the work of other resident artists and craftsmen that was sold to benefit a building drive.

His interest in aviation brought many invitations for airplane rides and meetings with famous aviators of the 1930s and 1940s, including Wiley Post. "In 1930, when the first autogyro was flown over the Lehigh Valley by the Silverbrook Coal Co. of Bethlehem, Papa Raker and I were aboard," Eric recalled.

When he died in 1982, Eric had been at the Home longer than any other resident.

Eric and his art work made the cover of *Sweet Charity* repeatedly. But perhaps the most touching was for the January-February 1939 issue where Eric was shown receiving art lessons.

Below the photo was a letter from Laura B. Watts of

Elkins Park to Papa Raker, praising the Home for opening the door to those who know not where to go. She wrote, "The case of Eric Andrews has always been one of life's miracles."

* * *

The board minutes of August 11, 1911, say tersely: "William Remaley, Parryville, was received."

He was seven, paralyzed with infantile paralysis. He hopped about like a frog on all fours. But whether it was by wheelchair, wagon or his crawling, he made his way. He was hauled to Jefferson School in a wagon in the beginning.

He also had the special distinction of being a babysitter for Connie Raker. "And I still have the scars to prove it," Connie would jokingly say over the years.

In 1919, Papa Raker took Bill and Charles Schilling to be examined by a noted surgeon in Philadelphia and then to be admitted to Episcopal Hospital for corrective surgery. "I was in the hospital seventeen weeks," Bill recalls.

It wasn't long before he was learning to walk with crutches and braces. The crutches would be for speed.

And as that 1924 item in Papa's report to the board revealed, Bill Remaley was starting a career with The Good Shepherd Home laundry that would go until his retirement in 1979. For fifty-three years, he served as supervisor of that facility.

Early on also, Papa Raker sent him to business college for a while.

In 1943, he married Grace Ernst, who had come to the Home two years earlier and wound up a nurses aide for forty-three years. "They gave me a home because at that time I needed one," Grace says.

"Conrad married us," Bill says.

Now in joint retirement, they reside in a house Good Shepherd owns just a block away from the main complex. His getting about now is strictly by wheelchair. "Since I retired, my legs gave out," he explains.

Bill has been around Good Shepherd so long that as a kid he saw the houses go up on the south side of St.

156

John Street and now is seeing some of them come down.

* * *

As Papa said in his note to the board, the Ahner children—Eva, Luther and Ella—were a special case.

Their mother, Lizzie, was one of the first girls admitted to the Topton Orphan Home. "She was like a daughter to us, and we were like parents to her," said Papa of those Topton Home years.

First the father became ill and then the mother. It was natural for Lizzie to turn to Mama and Papa Raker. At one point, the whole family was at Good Shepherd.

Then the father died and Lizzie realized she had little time left. Her abiding concern was the care and Christian training of her three little children. She begged Papa to assume the responsibility for their bodies and souls. He said he would do all he could, and that to him was a sacred promise.

Already in 1925, *Sweet Charity* was hailing achievements for all three Ahner children:

"Eva is doing good work in high school and after graduation next year will enter the Normal School and prepare for teaching. Luther passed the Twelfth Ward grade school for high school without examination and the highest praises of the principal. Ella won the five-dollar prize for the best essay, 'On a Trip to the Allen Laundry,' in the freshman class of the Allentown High School in the domestic science course."

Papa, of course, ran Ella's essay in *Sweet Charity*.

The sacred promise was being kept.

* * *

Verna Hoppes, the farm girl from near Tamaqua, had quite a chapter of her life to unfold as she addressed thousands at the 1934 Anniversary Day program.

"No doubt, you have often seen my picture and heard about me, but perhaps you have never heard the story from my own lips.

"When I was born, I was a healthy, normal child. I romped and played like all of you have done and

157

perhaps are yet doing.

"But when I was eight, the great misfortune came upon me of losing the advantage of my lower limbs, just by the mere trampling into a nail. I was taken from hospital to hospital where various operations were performed, thus giving me the job of being able to walk with the aid of crutches and braces.

"As the years went by, I was led to the doors of The Good Shepherd Home. Here, I was to get an education, also a religious education and vision. Here, I found friends who so willingly stood by me and helped me. Here, I learned to carry my cross with a smile.

"When I entered the Home, I was almost helpless and, perhaps, just as hopeless. My first year of school was spent under the tutorship of Rev. Oscar Minkus.

"Finally my strength permitted me to go to public school. So as the years went by, I reached the first goal in life I had set for myself—to graduate from the Allentown High School.

"I have new visions and hope for the future. If it is God's will and nothing interferes, I will enter Cedar Crest College this fall."

Four years later, she was before the Anniversary Day audience again, this time with her Cedar Crest diploma and a job.

"After the crippled body has been educated, the greatest problem of all presents itself—the employment problem," said Verna.

"People in all walks of life eagerly applaud and utter words of admiration when they hear of the educational progress made by a handicapped person. But are they anxious to furnish employment for them?

"No! Just as soon as the businessman sees the crutches, it is graciously stated, 'We don't have anything for you now, but come around later.'

"My friends, that so-called later never comes.

"Today, I bow in gratitude that there is one man in the world who has not turned me down because of my condition. Mr. George M. Sowers, two days after my commencement from Cedar Crest College, employed me as the official secretary in the Allentown Agency of the Lutheran Brotherhood Insurance Co.

"Would to God that the world had more men that were broad-minded and of the same caliber as Mr. Sowers, because then the employment problem of the handicapped person would be solved."

Papa would report to the board that Verna won prizes in history and accounting at commencement. "The Good Shepherd Home was never more honored than on this occasion. We recommend the Home acknowledge the marked attention and great kindness the faculty and the students of Cedar Crest College showed towards our handicapped girl."

And there would be other glorious chapters in this woman's life.

*   *   *

Raymond Myers, the first armless boy at the Home, became a photo personality in *Sweet Charity*. He was shown playing a guitar or the piano with his toes.

He was the first armless person with a driver's license in Pennsylvania, and *Sweet Charity* published a copy of the letter from the state's motor vehicle agency verifying that.

Ray achieved fame by being cited in Ripley's Believe It or Not. And he performed in 1934 at the Ripley Odditorium at the Chicago World's Fair.

*   *   *

George Goldfus would eclipse Eric Andrews' longevity record at Good Shepherd.

To recognize that, the Home chose George as the first one to cross the walkway high over South Sixth Street to his new home in the Conrad W. Raker Center. The event was the cover of the September-October 1980 issue of *Sweet Charity*, with George all smiles in his motorized wheelchair.

To quote George from an earlier time in *Sweet Charity*: "We hope that our friends of The Good Shepherd Home will remember us in their prayers and know that they are most appreciated for making possible all these blessings here at the Home."

*   *   *

These glimpses into the lives of some Good Shepherd residents preach the cause in their own way—just as Papa preached in his. Please permit two further living parables by Papa to close out this chapter:

Near the end of his life, Papa told about a sour rich man, Herman L. Willig of Lancaster, who was left all alone. His attitude was that he cared for no one and nobody seemed to care for him. In prosperous days, he made no friends and when he became old, he was left without a friend.

A fellow minister told Papa that Willig had inquired about The Good Shepherd Home. Papa went to see him.

Willig asked: "What are your boarding terms per month?"

Papa: "The Good Shepherd Home is not a boarding house, but a Home, right now filled to overflowing. Age, faithfulness and need are especially taken into consideration when we do have room. And deserving ones who have no money are taken in."

As Papa saw the situation, this man thought because he had money, some poor person should be pushed aside and the room given to him.

Synod subsequently met in Lancaster, and despite predictions from board member Solomon E. Ochsenford that Papa could do Willig no good and that the man would not do anything for Good Shepherd, Papa went to see him again.

Willig finally went to a home for old people, and that didn't suit him. He got sick and was put in a hospital, and he was displeased with the way the hospital was run.

Papa got an earful when he saw Willig at the hospital. Willig accused Papa of not visiting him at the old folks home where he had been staying for six months.

Willig attacked The Good Shepherd Home. "You are not honest. You promised to take the most needy. But when I wanted to enter, even if I had money, you made no attempt to receive me. I don't want anything to do with The Good Shepherd Home anymore."

Here was an opportunity for Papa to take Apostolic leave—shaking the dust from his feet from the room of this miserable man and departing.

But instead, he boldly stepped to the bed and prayed over Willig:

"O God, the Father in Heaven, for Jesus sake, have mercy upon this poor, sick, benighted, unhappy soul of Thine, whom Thou didst redeem with Thy most precious blood, but who has forgotten his baptismal vow, his confirmation vow and forgotten Thee and Thy Church and here lies, on the borders of time and eternity, unable to move, with one foot in the grave.

"O, we pray Thee, Blessed Jesus, let Thine infinite mercy, love and compassion lead him to true repentance and faith in Thee, while Thou art near, or before his day of grace be ended, the door be shut and his poor soul be lost forever and forever. Amen."

Papa then recited the Old and New Testament benedictions, said "I now leave you alone with God" and quickly left for fear he would be ordered out. He never saw Willig again.

To Papa's great surprise, the man put a codicil in his will giving Good Shepherd $7,200 without a string to it.

"We expect to meet him in heaven," Papa said later, "not because he gave this money to the Home, but because we have reasons to believe he confessed his sin and was forgiven. Life from the dead, so let it be. Amen!"

*　*　*

Dr. Henry Trumbauer of Coopersburg was in St. Luke's Hospital in Bethlehem in 1929, nearing ninety and in failing health. And Papa had stopped by to see him on several occasions. "He appreciates the visits," Papa told the board. "I am his only spiritual adviser."

And the apparent reason for that was some long-standing disagreement between this physician and the Rev. William W. Kistler, the Lutheran pastor in Coopersburg. Whatever the cause, it had lasted more than twenty years.

Somehow, with Dr. Trumbauer dying, Papa got Rev.

Kistler to the doctor's hospital room.

"We did not know just what to do and decided to take a bold attitude," Papa later reported to the board. "We grasped Dr. Trumbauer's hand and Rev. Kistler's hand and offered a prayer, emphasizing the necessity of forgiving if we want to be forgiven."

Dr. Trumbauer said, "Brother Kistler, let us forgive one another all our sins and misunderstandings."

Rev. Kistler responded in the same beautiful spirit. Papa gave them Communion, and then Rev. Kistler said the benediction.

Papa turned to the dying man, "I'll continue to come see you sometimes. But from now on, Rev. Kistler will visit you as your pastor." ❖

Your old men shall dream
dreams, Your young men
shall see visions.

Joel 2:28

Conrad Weiser Raker says there was no shattering
event that led him to become the second
superintendent of The Good Shepherd Home. No
lightning striking. No burning bush on the road to
Damascus.

"I was sort of led into it," Connie says. "My father
had a lot to do with that.

"At seminary, I loved to go out and preach. There
was some congregation out in Berks County that was
interested in me. But Papa said to just wait a bit."

With Connie's graduation from Philadelphia
Lutheran Seminary in the spring of 1937, the board of
The Good Shepherd Home asked him to be the Home's
assistant superintendent. He readily accepted.

Papa was in his mid-seventies and still sharp
mentally as his words in *Sweet Charity* attest. But he
was ailing physically. Giving him an assistant
superintendent was a caring way to go about what
would soon be the end of his reign. The board put
Papa's feelings uppermost.

Connie served as assistant until Papa's death in May
1941. Two months later, the board named him
superintendent. His title would be changed to
administrator in 1967. But whatever the title, he ran

Good Shepherd either under his father or on his own for forty-three years.

He would put Good Shepherd on the map for its work in rehabilitation and employment of the handicapped. And even in retirement after 1980, he would be adored and almost worshipped by those touched by what he has done.

The great joy of serving Good Shepherd was the personal relationship with the residents, Connie says. "I see people in wheelchairs all crippled up and think, 'Raker, if you were like that, you'd be miserable.' I walked outside one day to a group of a half dozen people in their wheelchairs on the front patio at Raker Center. It was a beautiful day, and one of those wheelchair people remarked, 'Isn't it a great day to be alive.'

"I've lived among heroes, and I mean that."

Connie is a very different person from his father—a private individual in many ways compared to the lay-it-all-on-the-line approach of Papa's . . . a tall, almost shy man compared to that feisty bantam rooster of a father.

Yet, each seems to be most appropriate for the era of Good Shepherd that he served . . . Papa the rough and tumble pioneer clearing the land for what he called the most helpless of humanity, Connie the one to cultivate that cleared land into a place where they could grow and thrive.

Both possessed a deep understanding of human need. Both were motivated by a strong Christian faith. And, as a result, both were capable of moving mountains.

The ancient Greeks divided mankind rather ruthlessly into two classes—Greeks and barbarians. If you were a Greek, you were all right. If you were a barbarian, you just didn't belong.

The children of The Good Shepherd Home had a little of the spirit of the ancient Greeks. Either you were a "Home boy" or an "outsider."

Many of the children of the Home knew exactly when they arrived and how long they were there. Connie, while still a child, once innocently asked his mother: "How long have I been at the Home?"

Connie was a Home boy, born October 27, 1912, the only manchild of John H. and D. Estella (Weiser) Raker to survive beyond infancy. He was baptized by Dr. Wackernagel.

He came into the world with two sisters and an extended family then numbering forty orphans and six old people.

At age two, he was accorded the place of honor to lead the Christmas procession of young and old into the parlor of the Kline homestead to behold the decorated tree and the filled stockings for each person.

On Connie's fifth birthday in 1917, Papa took the whole family to the seminary at Mt. Airy for the unveiling of a monument to Henry Melchior Muhlenberg, the patriarch of the Lutheran Church in America.

Papa told *Sweet Charity* readers: "We were especially interested in the erection of this monument because our children claim to be direct descendants of Muhlenberg. (If Muhlenberg had been a questionable character, we would not press the claim.)

"Muhlenberg was married to a daughter of the distinguished Indian agent, Conrad Weiser, the first judge of Berks County, Pennsylvania.

"We wanted all our children to be present at the unveiling. October 27 was the fifth birthday of our son, Conrad Weiser Raker, and we were especially anxious that he should be so impressed with the fact that he will remember the unveiling when he attends the seminary at Mt. Airy."

It was obvious that Papa was already doing some leading.

And when Connie was only ten, he was a member of the band, a trumpet player, for its trip through the coal regions and Papa's childhood area of Northumberland County. As Clarence Nissley, the Home's noted writer, recorded:

"We also went on the Isle of Que at Selinsgrove, which Shickalimy, the Indian chief, presented to Conrad Weiser, the great Indian interpreter. The superintendent and son slept on the isle."

Connie's sister Ruth was along on the band trip as the girl's caretaker. But it was Connie who would get the full lesson in family history.

Connie was just one of four "Good Shepherd Home boys" confirmed on Palm Sunday 1927 by the Rev. Phares Beer at Grace Lutheran Church. The four were on the cover of the May-June 1927 *Sweet Charity* in their Sunday best. Simply: "Names left to right: Gerald Guinn, Earl Walbert, Stephen Oller and Conrad Weiser Raker."

Connie went to Allentown schools, as did just as many of the Home children as were able. He was in the crew to harvest the crops on the Home farm, just as the other children of the Home. As he grew, he helped with the summer camp for the Home boys along the banks of the Little Lehigh.

When a high school senior, he developed a bad case of bronchitis, so severe that a doctor in the neighborhood recommended that Papa and Mama send him to Saranac, the famed tuberculosis sanitarium in upstate New York, to recuperate. There was no sign of TB, the doctor assured.

Papa asked: "How much is it going to cost?"

The doctor: "Five hundred dollars."

Papa: "I can't afford it."

The doctor: "You beg, borrow or steal it."

Connie went—for six weeks. It was long enough to cut into his schoolwork at Allentown High, so he finished instead at Allentown Prep.

He still considers himself a member of the Class of 1930 at Allentown High and is called upon to give the invocation at class reunions.

Papa loved to hunt. And he devoted the whole back cover of a 1932 *Sweet Charity* to 1931 hunting scenes at the Black Wolf Rod and Gun Club of Liberty, Pennsylvania. This included a picture of Connie, "after shooting his first deer December 1, 1931," posing flanked by the carcasses of two deer hanging from a tree limb.

Sweet Charity proclaimed: "We know of no physical culture or exercise that will promote health, strength and purity in a boy or young man like hunting in the

166

pure mountain air of the pine-clad primal forests of good old Pennsylvania. We know of nothing that will rejuvenate a man when his breath becomes short and the joints become stiff like hunting and worshipping God in His first temples, the groves."

One *Sweet Charity* reader from Germantown—a former Sunday school pupil of Papa's—wrote to tell him that cover layout was nauseating. She asked: How could a humanitarian like him, one who sets such a Christian example, encourage young boys to hunt, saying it is a worthy sport? What of the cruelty of the thing, the wounded birds and animals crawling away to die in agony?

When Connie read the letter, he said, "There is a great deal of truth in it."

Papa added, "It is practically all truth."

And, of course, Papa ran the letter in *Sweet Charity* along with his response.

Papa said he always tried to keep his heart pure, warm and tender. Man was created to have dominion over all God's creatures, and these creatures are for our use, certainly not to be abused and tortured.

"We believe the wild game is intended for man. Of the thousands of deer that were shot, many were given to hospitals and The Good Shepherd Home has always received more than its portion of those that were illegally shot."

(For years, Papa had openly solicited on the pages of *Sweet Charity* the contraband of illegally killed deer seized by game protectors and thanked those protectors who sent them to the Home.)

Papa's response continued: "Now these wild animals cannot be secured like chickens and cattle in the barnyard. We believe, however, that great care should be taken by hunters so as not to cripple or cause unnecessary suffering."

And, of course, Papa could not tell a story without working in some application to Good Shepherd. This instance was no exception. He concluded:

"We have always tried to encourage kindness to animals and birds. We have had a number of specialists come to The Good Shepherd Home and lecture to our children on this subject.

"When Governor Gifford Pinchot gave his consent to hunt doe in certain counties last fall, he did so because they were so plentiful that many would have starved to death during the winter, which would have been much more cruel than the shooting.

"Growing boys must be occupied in something that will interest them to keep them out of mischief. Personally, I have found nothing that helped me (and my boys) more, physically and spiritually, than to roam in the pure mountain air, near to nature and God's nature."

Connie is an alumnus of Muhlenberg College, Class of 1934. Much as Papa proclaimed the academic achievements of the boys and girls of the Home, *Sweet Charity* said nothing about Connie in his college years.

The only item was something Connie wrote himself, briefly citing the responsibilities of being manager of the Muhlenberg debating team, "the most abused and maltreated person on the squad." More extensively, he hailed the work of the coach, Arthur T. Gillespie. "Undoubtedly to Art more than one student owes his success at law school."

It was to be typical of Connie, only lightly mentioning his own involvement as a springboard to sing the praises of others.

At graduation, *Sweet Charity* simply carried the photos of the Home's three boys who were in Muhlenberg's Class of 1934—Clarence Putt, Harry Filer and Conrad W. Raker. No special treatment for the superintendent's kid.

Connie is a graduate of the Lutheran Theological Seminary at Mt. Airy, Class of 1937.

While at seminary, he took additional night courses at the Wharton School of Finance at the University of Pennsylvania. He also helped at the Germantown Home for the aged during his senior year.

He was ordained May 19, 1937, at St. Andrew's by the Sea in Atlantic City at the annual gathering of the Lutheran Ministerium.

"My son, Conrad, is preparing himself for institutional work," Papa told the Good Shepherd board just before it extended Connie a call.

In announcing Connie as assistant superintendent, Papa told *Sweet Charity* readers:

"During his early youth, Conrad showed special consideration toward the feelings of others. This is the fundamental necessity for success in the work of the Master, especially in this age when needs are measured by cold numbers rather than souls and social work is considered something solely an object of legislation and not a challenge of the cardinal Christian precept—Love."

Connie began his work that June 1 with great enthusiasm, Papa wrote. "We feel sure that he will continue throughout his life to do all within his power to help those who have none to help them."

Papa said a bit more in his report at that time to the board: "Conrad has done better than I expected, which shows that I did not expect enough. He must increase and I must decrease. May the increase be rapidly and the decrease slowly."

Connie had intended to spend a year in Europe in special preparation for this work. But the trustees suggested it would be better to study the institutions of America first. He was taking a special course at Temple University in connection with work outlined by Dr. Gustavus "Gus" Bechtold, secretary of the Lutheran Inner Mission Bureau.

"All wish him God's blessing in his chosen work," Papa said in concluding the announcement in *Sweet Charity*. "He is presenting the Good Shepherd Home cause in different churches nearly every Sunday. Write for dates."

Ah, yes, "Write for dates." How delightfully typical of Papa—using every opportunity to peddle The Good Shepherd Home—even in the announcement of his own son's hiring.

Connie was installed that August 8 in St. Michael's Lutheran Church in Allentown by the Rev. Dr. Conrad Wilker, president of the Allentown Conference of the Ministerium of Pennsylvania and also president of the board of trustees of The Good Shepherd Home.

And it was also Dr. Wilker who introduced Connie to

the crowd at the twenty-ninth Anniversary Day just four days later:

"Pastor Conrad Raker is well qualified, especially because of his fine appreciation of the great possibilities and opportunities that lie before our Home and challenge our best efforts as one of the truly great agencies of the Church."

Connie responded that in the three months he was already at work he was seeing things a bit differently than he did as a student.

It's horrifying but tempting to become bogged down in detail work from morning to evening, he told the gathering. "Living in such an endless procession of days we lose sight of the things of higher value.

"We must ever keep in mind the cause of the crippled and needy child, not simply view our work as a task to be done, but as a part of the great work of the Church of Christ," Connie said.

Hard as the work may be, already there are rewards, Connie said.

He cited William Clapper, a Home boy who had just finished high school and was going on to college, who spoke from the same platform earlier in the day.

"During the course of his talk, he said, 'Because of my training at The Good Shepherd Home I now view my life as an opportunity for service.' To hear that boy say that and to know full well he meant it is one of the great rewards for work at The Good Shepherd Home."

He ended with a promise to all the friends of the Home:

"I pledge to the work of The Good Shepherd Home all of my energy, that the crippled, the neglected, the handicapped might be taken better care of, that they might be better prepared to meet life and that this Home may truly carry on as it has begun—that it will be the true Shepherd of the souls within its care."

Shortly after Connie took on his work, Papa confessed to *Sweet Charity* readers that he had had his first and only sickness. He called it "depression." The result was that the Home's cause was not personally presented in the churches by Papa for more than a year.

"Thank the Lord we are now getting over it and are ready to sow by all waters. The assistant superintendent is now preparing for a greater Good Shepherd Home. He will also be able to give some of his time to present the cause."

Preparing for a greater Good Shepherd Home in part meant a year of taking courses at both Temple University and the University of Pennsylvania—courses in social work.

Good heavens, Papa's son taking courses in social work! Papa had vilified social workers for years across the pages of *Sweet Charity*. They were those folks who felt the churches ought to get out of the social welfare business and let the state handle it all.

One of them even breezed into town from the State Welfare Department some years earlier to tell Papa he was doing a pretty good job, but—to improve—he should have the children weighed every day. Papa responded that the workers at Good Shepherd had a lot more important things to do than weigh the children daily.

But it was obvious from the reports Connie was sending back to the board he was learning things that would help at Good Shepherd.

He attended a panel discussion dealing with case studies involving two youngsters in industrial schools. "I found myself forgetting that these children were delinquent court cases and applying the same therapeutic methods of social rehabilitation to several of our own children at the Home.

"The value of approaching the individual from many different fields is obvious. There were on the panel doctors, case workers, psychiatrists, psychologists and a specialist in the field of education."

At the Home for Incurables at Byberry he had a long talk with the supervisor on the handling, washing and educating of these children. "A great phase of our work is becoming more and more the care of incurables," Connie observed.

He was also reading case histories and going out in the field as a case worker for the Lutheran Children's Bureau.

"The bureau takes great care in writing these histories," he wrote to the board. "Family conditions are investigated. Foster homes are thoroughly examined before a placement is made, and then all is written into the files so that at any later date a complete picture of the child's history may be had.

"Of all the impressions made upon me, the greatest is the need at our Home for an excellent system of individual case records." Without criticizing Papa's administration, he was gently saying some things were going to be different under him.

At the end of the 1937-38 academic year, Connie said his return to the actual duties at the Home gave greater importance to the courses he had taken in social work, the administration of social agencies and such.

"While studying these courses, I felt much of what was discussed in class was either trite or so radical that either way you looked at it, it was foolish. Now, I look with a more kindly eye at the things discussed in some of these courses."

Much of his time had been spent in field work for the Board of Inner Missions—visiting with prison and hospital chaplains and supervising fifteen boys of the Lutheran Children's Bureau, then writing case histories on them that traced their progress.

He repeated his original assertion that the best lesson for him was the importance of keeping individual records. He and office secretary Winifred Hammer had already begun a thorough revision of Good Shepherd records—including adding a face sheet that listed the highlights of each child's life.

During the course of the year, Dr. Bechtold had sent him to several social service conferences. "These were always conducted by progressive people in the realm of social service, and while many of them have no regard for the organized work of the Church, still there is much for us to learn from them."

At one such conference, Dr. Carl DeSchweinitz said that the social work by private institutions—the great pioneers in this field—would continue as energetically and useful as ever.

Connie had visited numerous institutions and read extensively.

"The personal interest of Dr. Bechtold has been a great asset in giving me a view of the work as a whole. Many times, not only in staff conference meetings but in private, he has discussed the social problems of the Church."

He concluded, "All these factors have contributed toward a clear vision of my work."

Papa was forty-five with the experience of two parishes and the work of the Topton Orphanage behind him when he started Good Shepherd with one youngster.

Connie was in his mid-twenties when he took on much of the responsibility of the Home, with a population of about seventy children and thirty old folks, to help his ailing father and twenty-nine when that responsibility was all his. ❖

Where there is no vision, the people perish.

Proverbs 29:18

"The Lutherans have always been too modest to let their light shine," *Sweet Charity* of November-December 1938 accused. It was an accusation Papa had voiced almost since the first day The Good Shepherd Home was operating.

Sweet Charity even told that message once in a poem called "Publicity." It went:

> One step won't take you very far,
> You've got to keep on walking;
> One word won't tell folks who you are,
> You've got to keep on talking;
> One inch won't make you very tall,
> You've got to keep on growing;
> One little ad won't do it all,
> You've got to keep 'em going.

Papa had *Sweet Charity* to let the Home's light shine. He had the local newspapers and even the ones beyond the immediate area carry the message of the Home, often publishing word for word Papa's material the way he sent it in.

He had that one zany promotion in 1919 of dropping leaflets and copies of *Sweet Charity* from an airplane to advertise that year's Anniversary Day. He preached the cause in the churches throughout the area and beyond. He preached it from courthouse steps and in public parks on the band tours.

When radio came along in the early 1920s, he was broadcasting the cause from a local station and had the youngsters from the Home singing, reading and otherwise performing on it.

"I heard you on the radio" was the expression Papa was getting from all directions in the mid-1920s from those who heard him on the first Friday of the month at 8:15 p.m. on WCBA, the Queen City Radio Broadcasting Station. Listeners sent donations. Others asked for copies of *Sweet Charity*.

The joke was: Give Papa any Bible text and he'd somehow manage to work it around to The Good Shepherd Home.

And William Pitten, the boy with the crutch in the strawberry patch with the Pauley sisters, built one of the first radio sets in Allentown right at the Home.

Papa arranged to have Pitt show off his contraption to the members of the advisory board and the trustees as a prelude to their meeting.

The radio didn't work. Pitt made adjustments. It still didn't work. Papa finally said, "Well, William, we must get down to business. You play with your set somewhere else."

Pitt picked up his radio and left, his head lowered, his hour of triumph transformed into embarrassment.

The men were deep into business discussion when suddenly the door flew open and there stood Pitt, smiling broadly and shouting, "It works. It works."

Papa was horrified. But the board members quickly gathered around to hear Pitt's radio. "They were dumbfounded, completely dumbfounded," Pitt recalled.

Papa wasn't quite as impressed. Later that day, he gave Pitt a spanking. Radio or no radio, he shouldn't have broken into the board meeting.

Papa invited pre-theological students from Muhlenberg College and seminary students from Mt. Airy and Gettysburg theological schools to come for a tour and a chicken dinner—figuring that once they got out in their congregations, they would help spread the message of Good Shepherd.

And he knew then what advertising in every media tells us every day. You repeat your message, again and again and again, to make sure it gets through.

Almost from the start of his career, Connie planned a giant step beyond all those means Papa had used. He dreamed of a movie.

He reported to the board in September 1939, "For some time, we have been contemplating a motion picture which will tell the world of the Home. John Kohl, the Sunday editor of *The Morning Call*, has promised to write the scenario."

He had already spoken to people at the Lutheran Publication House and gotten hints on how to go about this. A theatrical group called Play and Players from Bethlehem had promised its support.

Connie asked the board: "Is it possible to do this?

"The plan in mind is to tell the life stories of four children who came to the Home, picture their growth and the advantages and opportunities given by the Home.

"This would have a great contact value in presenting the cause."

The board, acknowledging this would be a project that would take some time, immediately endorsed it.

Connie was back to the board again about a year later with more on the movie idea. At the Omaha Convention of what was then the United Lutheran Church in America, he had gotten a suggestion from the Lutheran Film Service to contact Willard Pictures in New York City.

He did. And Willard Pictures showed him movies made for the Boys Club of America and the Mil-Bank, a summer home for boys and girls from the slums. He felt both told their stories well. Lowell Thomas, world traveler and probably the most famous newscaster of the day, was the narrator for the one, Raymond Graham Swing for the other.

Connie also visited News Reel Laboratory in Philadelphia, a smaller operation where he came away with what he felt were two particularly good ideas: Make a short picture with a news commentator describing the action you see with that voice crisp and clearcut and, secondly, once you have a dynamic picture like that, national theater distribution is an easy matter for a small fee.

In February 1941, the board entered into a contract with Willard Pictures for a total of $4,000 and the subsequent delivery of "one 16mm reduction print."

Within weeks, the firm had decided on Lowell Thomas, who graciously volunteered his services.

After he was fully acquainted with the work of caring for those who are physically handicapped at The Good Shepherd Home, Lowell Thomas interrupted with the exclamation, "Why, this is a home in every sense of the word, not an institution. The children can even invite their neighborhood friends home for dinner."

To Connie, nothing that had ever been said about Good Shepherd had pleased him so much as that comment.

And at Connie's behest, Willard Pictures was to hold off filming until a little later in the year "so the beauty of the surroundings would show at its very best." Willard Pictures agreed.

As Connie reported to the board in early June, "The actual taking of the motion picture has again been postponed. The picture will be taken the week of June 30.

"Unfortunately, some changes will have to be made. My father was to have been photographed in the picture."

Papa Raker had died May 8, 1941. *The New York Times* as well as newspapers throughout Good Shepherd's immediate area carried his obituary. His funeral was a major event in Allentown, and the accolades for his achievements were once again proclaimed far and wide.

The filming of the picture went on during the week of June 30 as planned. A photo of Papa was shown on a table as the camera zoomed in and Papa's founding work was extolled. "Conrad has taken his father's responsibility on his shoulders," Lowell Thomas explained.

As Connie saw it, the picture would be a wonderful

advertisement for the Home. He was right.

It was called "Because Somebody Cares." It made its theater debut at the Colonial in Allentown March 5, 1942, with "Mr. Bug Goes to Town," billed as the happiest full-length feature cartoon ever filmed, starring Honey and Hoppity. If the feature film had any significance in theater history, it may be for the song, "I'll Dance at Your Wedding."

The Colonial in its nearly quarter-page newspaper ad heralding the arrival of the film said not a word about The Good Shepherd Home short to run with it.

Connie was less than happy that "Because Somebody Cares" ran with what he called such a poor feature film. But it was soon to go to other theaters in town. More important, all the comments coming back were favorable.

It began with Lowell Thomas winding up a regular news broadcast, including his famous line: "And so long until tomorrow."

The microphone is removed and Thomas starts talking informally about how democracy and Christianity are inseparable, that both consider the development of the individual essential.

Then, he mentions that in Allentown, Pennsylvania, there is an institution called The Good Shepherd Home that is making the brotherhood of man a living reality and is truly expressing Christian democracy.

"The only requirement is real need," Lowell Thomas explained. And those in need will find help in good measure at Good Shepherd, he said.

The film showed a family living in a shack. "The mother is a mental case. The father is just no good," Thomas intoned. The dirty and disheveled children had to sleep on a mattress on the floor.

One boy from that family, however, is taken to The Good Shepherd Home. He is cleaned up. He is sent to the public school with the other boys of the Home. He is on his way to a worthwhile life.

Most important, the film said, was the care of crippled children. The message was that most became self-reliant.

There were scenes of Eric Andrews studying art . . .

Morris Blinderman working to become a writer . . . the infant Martin Revelette, the armless boy, holding his bottle with his feet.

Also, there were pictures of Verna Hoppes, who was graduated from Cedar Crest College in 1938; Harry Filer, the Home's Caruso who was Muhlenberg College Class of 1934; Clarence Nissley, the Home's Horace Greeley who was Muhlenberg College 1931, Mt. Airy Seminary 1934 and then a graduate student at Columbia University.

Raymond Myers, the first armless boy to grow up at the Home, was shown driving his car.

As Connie told *Sweet Charity* readers: "For those who have followed the activities of The Good Shepherd Home, much will be familiar. You will recognize the children. You will recognize the boys and girls who have grown to manhood and womanhood and are now earning their own living."

The film immediately became a part of Connie's presentation when he went out to churches and other groups to explain the cause.

Arranging for national or even regional distribution in theaters was something else again, especially in wartime.

Connie traveled to New York in mid-1942 to see about theatrical distribution. What he learned was that the government was making so many short subjects dealing with the war and giving them to the individual theaters for free that the theaters were no longer finding it necessary to buy short subjects.

"If a picture doesn't have a war angle, it doesn't seem very welcome," Connie reported to the board. "We tried to explain to the different men with whom we spoke that a picture like ours is a very good one for frayed war nerves. All the men who saw our picture were well pleased with it."

One distributor asked five dollars from the Home for each theater he got the film into, regardless of how long it ran.

The YMCA Distribution Center said if the Home provided twenty copies, it would guarantee a quarter million people a year would see the picture. Their regular charge was seventy-five dollars a print. For a charity like Good Shepherd, that fee would be twenty-five dollars.

"This seems very fair to me," Connie advised the board.

The YMCA Distribution Center was given ten prints, starting its showings in Brooklyn. It was an arrangement that would be continued for several years.

And Lowell Thomas said it would be fine to use his picture on a fund-raising brochure the Home was mailing out, along with the quote:

"What particularly appeals to me about The Good Shepherd Home is that the only requirement for admission is real need, regardless of money, creed, color or nationality. Any human being who needs help will find it here in good measure."

A couple years later, Connie was passing Allentown High School when the thought struck him that the boys and girls leaving the building would soon be men and women out in the community.

He went to the principal, then to the superintendent and readily secured permission to show "Because Somebody Cares" at an assembly program. He addressed the entire junior class and showed the picture at an assembly.

"I now plan to contact the various junior high schools of the city and show the picture there also," Connie told the board.

In late 1945, Connie reminded the trustees that the YMCA Bureau arrangement was indirect advertising, but still worthwhile.

"Several boys who recently returned from the service said they saw our picture at USO units and other places," he reported.

"Several years ago, the U.S. State Department asked to show 'Because Somebody Cares' in South America as part of the Good Neighbor Policy. We granted the permission, but heard nothing about it. We also granted permission to the Agriculture Department to use a certain scene from our picture in connection with special work they were doing."

The Home would once more turn to Lowell Thomas in 1948, this time for radio. A script writer named Don Russell, himself afflicted with infantile paralysis, wrote four five-minute scripts primarily for Lowell Thomas.

And Connie trooped to New York where he got a friendly reception from Lowell Thomas's secretary. The upshot was that Lowell Thomas did one of the scripts and assisted in getting other radio personalities to do the others.

Lowell Thomas donated his services as his way of contributing to the work of The Good Shepherd Home. For that, his was perhaps one of the most illustrious names partway down on a long list that extended back to 1908 to neighborhood shop keepers, local doctors and dentists, auxiliary members and potato farmers at New Tripoli.

B. Bryan Musselman of the Lehigh Valley Broadcasting Station made copies of the Lowell Thomas message. Connie gave them to local radio stations along with six one-minute spots.

They were distributed at the opportune time—just as the Christmas season approached. "We find that the donations from Allentown have greatly increased," Connie observed. "We think it is simply because of the fact they are reminded of it by radio."

There would be later filming, including:

—"Memories," two videos where Connie Raker and Carl Odhner did just what the title implies, share their recollections.

—"More than a Name . . . Good Shepherd," a 1982 film that outlined the contemporary work done in rehabilitation for people who need all kinds of healing.

—"Venture of Faith," an award-winning film produced by Robin Miller Filmaker in 1984 that featured a re-enactment of the funeral of tiny Viola Raker and the arrival of Viola Hunt in 1908 to start The Good Shepherd Home.

"Venture of Faith" has been shown as a short subject in commercial theaters in the Lehigh Valley—to 70,000 alone with the showing of Academy Award winning "Amadeus." There are also tapes of these that people can view on their VCRs at home.

Beyond that have been recent productions on people who have been honored by Good Shepherd, particularly those who have been named to the Handicapped Hall of Fame at Good Shepherd. These films show the achievements of the individuals in their everyday life as well as scenes from the program where they were honored.

These latest efforts—in color, of course—make the black and white Lowell Thomas film something of a film relic. But what a magnificent relic.

In 1962, upon his twenty-fifth anniversary as a pastor and administrator at Good Shepherd, Connie reminisced about getting the services of Lowell Thomas for that first film:

"People often asked me how we got him to do it. The most difficult part was simply to get to see him. After we explained The Good Shepherd Home to him, he readily consented." ❖

17: WORLD WAR II AND AFTERMATH

The whole world is in darkness and The Good Shepherd Home is one of the shining lights in this darkness.

Conrad Raker
January 11, 1942

Connie Raker had the mantle of leadership of Good Shepherd placed upon him in the same year that America entered World War II. And that war had some massive and diverse effects upon the Home.

Three days after the Japanese attacked Pearl Harbor on December 7, 1941, Connie reported to the board:

"With the recent outbreak of war in the Pacific, our minds have been thinking of just what the future of The Good Shepherd Home will be.

"Is the war going to have a noticeable effect on us?

"We are convinced that it will have many effects upon us, both good and bad. With increased earning power a possible increase in income for our appeals can be expected. But the increase in taxes and the general business of carrying on the war may detract a great deal.

"We are personally convinced that in the new period into which we are going, we must go as conservatives, but not mossbacks . . . conservatives in that we waste nothing, but yet build progressively.

"Our facilities must be used to the utmost."

As Connie predicted, there were many effects of the

183

war, good and bad:

One of the Home's own boys, Staff Sgt. Robert Condus, was killed while on maneuvers in the service in Australia. In leaving for the military, that young man had named Connie his adopted brother to inherit what little he had should there be a reason to inherit. Bobby's death was devastating to those at the Home who had grown up with him. He was much loved.

The Home farm lost much of its acreage for the construction of an airfield and plant to make torpedo bombers for the Navy—only to see the project branded a giant waste. The Navy got just a handful of bombers for its $85 million. And the paving over what once was farmland quickly told the Good Shepherd trustees that no postwar reclamation was possible.

The Home became a refuge for various kinds of victims of the war—a doctor and his family who fled Nazi Germany before America entered the war . . . the wife and children of an Army chaplain who was away in the service . . . European refugees at the end of the war who needed a temporary home until they were located in permanent quarters . . . and Constantino Basile "Dino" Katsiaris, a Greek boy who had both hands blown away by a hand grenade in the unsuccessful effort by the Communists to take over the government in his homeland in the early years after the war.

If anyone symbolized the most that Good Shepherd could achieve, it was Dino. He was an in-house hero. And his life was closely followed in the pages of *Sweet Charity* for years.

At a later time, there would be Mennonite males who were conscientious objectors who labored at Good Shepherd as their alternative to military service.

In 1943, Connie himself tried to enlist in the Navy as a chaplain. He got as far as a first interview in Philadelphia. But when he went back a second time, his file had been pulled.

The Good Shepherd board had somehow intervened.

The board minutes of October 1943 reflect that President James F. Henninger and member G. Franklin Gehr had met with Connie to consider a

184

matter weighing heavily upon him—the urgent call by the government and the Lutheran Church for more Army and Navy chaplains and Connie's own inner promptings at age thirty to respond to such a call.

They said the discussion was frank. Their conclusion:

"In view of the many changes through which our Home is now passing . . . the many problems facing our Home during and after the war . . . the scarcity of capable leaders to take the place of our superintendent . . . the irreparable loss our Home might suffer in his absence, it was the judgment of the committee that the greater duty at this time was for him to remain with and serve the Home."

The committee left its decision open, should it appear later that the need for naval chaplains becomes "imperative."

It is a rather perverse fact that wars have done much to improve the way we save and restore those they have maimed and battered. It is the returning wounded warrior who receives the first and best of the new methods to try to make him whole again. But the benefits spill over to the institutions that serve the civilian population as well.

* * *

Bobby Condus was the first young man drafted from Good Shepherd and the first and only one to fall. He was born Sept. 4, 1919. He went to Jefferson Elementary and on to Allentown High, where he was a graduate with the Class of 1940. He spent virtually his entire life at the Home until late 1940 when he got a job at Western Electric and moved out of Good Shepherd. Then, he was drafted into the Army on March 1, 1941. A newly formed Good Shepherd Alumni Association held a farewell party for him.

Bobby's first assignment was Ft. Meade, Maryland, and Connie wrote a letter to the chaplain there, who happened to be a Lutheran, to look up Bobby.

Bobby's life had been pathetic. He was brought to the Home as a baby when his mother was apprehended in a police raid. He knew of no relatives at all.

Connie remembered a trip to Reading one time with Bobby along. They stopped at a store to make a small purchase.

As Connie turned to leave the store, he saw Bobby looking through the phone directory. Bobby's face colored as Connie asked, "Bobby, do you know anybody in Reading?"

"No," said Bobby. "But I want to see if anyone in Reading has the same name I do."

As Connie saw it, it was impossible for anyone who was more richly blessed to understand the depth of Bobby's wound of never knowing his actual family. Yet, he grew into manhood as a well-rounded individual.

As a boy and a man, Bobby was remembered for his friendliness, a friendliness that sprang from an inner concern for the welfare of others.

After the news of his death was announced to all the children and aged at Good Shepherd, a crippled boy on a wheelchair approached Connie and said, "I'll always have something to remind me of Bobby. When he was home on his last furlough, he bought me a guitar."

That act was typical of Bobby.

Bobby was killed November 16, 1943, in Camp Columbia at Queensland. The War Department notified Connie by telegram four days later.

What was rather haunting was that the Home subsequently received a Christmas card from Bobby, postmarked the day after his death.

But then shortly afterward a letter arrived from Bobby's chaplain, saying his body had been laid to rest in an American cemetery in Australia. "The presence of the officers and men of his unit and the number of floral pieces attested to the high esteem in which he was held by his comrades." The serial number mentioned was Bobby's.

Bobby left his adopted brother $10,000 in insurance and eight war bonds. Connie said they should go to the building fund.

And a year later, Rose Manson of Ipswich,

Queensland, Australia, wrote Connie a note:

"I thought you would like to know that someone in far away Australia is caring for the grave of your loved one, Robert Condus. Our garden overlooks the little cemetery, and in appreciation for all your boys have done for us, the token of flowers is the least I can give to express my own personal gratitude."

When Bobby died, there were twenty-three young men from the Home in the service, including eleven overseas.

In 1947, the War Department contacted Connie concerning the reburial of Bobby.

Connie had never agreed with those who felt American war dead should be returned to this country. So he filled out the forms and requested that the body "be interred in a permanent American Military Cemetery Overseas." For Bobby, that was to be the National Cemetery in Honolulu, then the Territory of Hawaii.

Bobby was the only Home boy to die in any American war.

* * *

The story of Dino Katsiaris is one that Connie seems to get so much joy in telling. And that probably had a lot to do with the fact that Dino was so fully followed in the pages of *Sweet Charity*.

The setting is post-war, but it really is a World War II story almost as much as Bobby Condus.

The Communists seemed to be succeeding in their fight to take over the governments in Greece and Turkey in the aftermath of the war. But President Truman and Secretary of State Dean Acheson sent American arms and military advisors to those nations. The tide was turned. The Communists were expelled.

Dino, a twelve-year-old in the Peloponnesian village of Kalamata whose mother had died when he was an infant, wound up a maimed victim of that fighting.

In June 1949, Dino and two friends had been called upon to carry a message to the government forces. They were asked because they were children and could get through when adults could not.

They made it and were on their way home when they were spotted by a Communist guerilla who threw a hand grenade. One boy lost an eye and the other was severely wounded in the stomach.

Dino bore almost the full brunt of the explosion. A leg was shattered in the blast, and when he tried to reach out to lean against a tree to help himself up, he realized his hands hung from his arms supported only by loose skin and lacerated flesh.

It was hours before he received medical help. The doctor removed Dino's hands.

The wife of the British ambassador to Greece took an interest in Dino and other children crippled as a result of the civil war. She arranged to have these children transported to England for further medical treatment.

Dino's uncle, a Greek national married to an American, wanted to bring Dino to this country. On June 16, 1950, the Congress of the United States voted that until June 30, 1951, a number of Greek displaced persons be allowed to enter the country. It opened the doors also for a certain number of children under sixteen. It opened the doors for Dino.

Connie Raker says the original inquiry to the Home about Dino came from a pastor in California. Then, the uncle contacted Good Shepherd. The board agreed to take him if the uncle made the necessary arrangements to get him into this country.

Dino arrived Oct. 24, 1951. He would touch the depths of love and compassion within Connie.

"We don't know when we can remember feeling as much sympathy for a boy as we did for this one, not alone for the nature of his handicapped condition, but also because he has been shunted around from one hospital to another and now finally has come to this country," Connie told the board.

Dino spoke no English when he arrived. He was a lonely boy. And there was a delay in enrolling him in school. So Connie took him along wherever he went on his daily rounds.

The first day, they returned too late for the noon meal at the Home. So Connie took him to his own house where Hannah prepared a lunch of soup and sandwiches. Dino just sat there and wouldn't eat.

Connie said, "Dino, please eat something so I can eat. I'm hungry." Dino smiled a bit and ate a few bites.

The next day, Connie took him to meet George Kalfas, the proprietor of the Superior Restaurant downtown, who also came from Greece. When Dino heard Greek spoken, his face lit up and a torrent of words poured out of this lonely boy.

Dino concedes the first few months at the Home were very unpleasant to him. "But I soon realized that The Good Shepherd Home was not really an institution as institutions go.

"One thing that really impressed me more than anything else was the relationship between the administrative staff and the guests. Although the guests varied in age, mental capacity, family background, etc., as far as the staff was concerned, all were equal before their eyes.

"In addition, I remember watching Dr. Raker closely in these early days, because he was the only one I exchanged my feelings with.

"I noticed one morning while Dr. Raker was coming from the chapel, he stopped and talked to all the people, young and old, and joked with them like he wasn't really the administrator.

"Then, I noticed that he stopped to talk with one person who had quite a low mental capacity. He was patient and talked with him for some time.

"With the constant help of Dr. Raker, I changed my attitude from one of gloominess to one of optimism."

The artificial hands Dino was using were of poor quality. The Home heard of remarkable work being done by Dr. Henry H. Kessler, founder of the Kessler Institute for Rehabilitation at West Orange, N.J.

Dr. Kessler had perfected a muscular operation known as cineplastic surgery, a tunneling done to the biceps. He had performed it on hundreds of GIs. Once the tunnel was healed, a piece of ivory half as long as a pencil was inserted into the tunnel. A piece of string was attached to the ivory.

The string was placed over a pulley attached to the end of the table. On the end of the string was tied a sandbag weighing five pounds. By contracting and relaxing the muscle, Dino raised and lowered the sandbag six or seven inches. This exercise prepared Dino for the artificial hand he was soon to receive.

Dino prospered. "In school, I began to realize there was a future for me if I worked hard. Work hard I did," he said.

Connie says it's rather beautiful the way one thing leads into another.

He was addressing the Parkway Manor Lions Club of Allentown in the spring of 1958, telling them some of the history of the Home and also something of the hopes and dreams for the future. He shared stories and incidents of the youngsters in his care.

At the end of the meeting, some members asked what they could do to help. Connie mentioned that Dino was being graduated that spring from Allentown High School. He desperately wanted to go to college.

They grasped the idea with a will and spoke to the entire club about it. The result was that a Lions club of twenty-two members sent Dino through Muhlenberg College. They paid everything—tuition, books, fees and other expenses. He was graduated in 1963.

Good Shepherd itself was able to send Dino on to Lehigh University for a master's degree in business administration in 1964. Lehigh gave him a partial scholarship. Good Shepherd made sure he had a single room so he could study.

When Dino was denied the chance to take a driver's test during his college years because of his artificial hands, he had the opportunity to present the matter directly to Governor David Lawrence when the governor visited the Home in 1961. Lawrence quickly straightened that out.

Since graduation from Lehigh, Dino has been an economist with the Veterans Administration in Washington. He served on Congressional committees on mortgage interest rates in 1969 that led to the deregulation of the savings and loan industry.

During the entire Carter administration, he briefed Veterans Administration director Max Cleland each Monday on economic and budget trends.

"I competed with people from Harvard, and I think I accounted for myself pretty well," he says.

He's in a $60,000-a-year-position involving loan guarantee service and mentions also that he's done well with investments.

Dino and Connie talk by phone twice a week. He stays with Connie and his wife, Grace, when he comes to Allentown. He calls Grace a warm person, a super lady.

Connie calls Dino a close personal friend.

Dino says that in his years at the Home, he and his contemporaries were all treated more or less the same. "Dr. Raker was generous with his time."

He calls Good Shepherd "really a home because of the interest. Even the staff, they were warm.

"I didn't know Papa Raker. But Mama Raker would always eat her meals with us. Those are the things that impress. It gave me a healthy outlook in life.

"From the guests to the people working there, they are a unique sort of people. I hope the spirit never dies.

"Dr. Raker was someone truly caring for you to succeed. He was showing an interest, a genuine interest, not just when the camera was there. He helped me gain confidence. He helped to get me where I am today.

"Few people will do the things Dr. Raker has done—not only for me, but for others.

"I will never forget."

* * *

Mennonites came to Good Shepherd at one point to perform alternate service. This was considerably after World War II. Perhaps more than what they did is what Connie saw in their presence at Good Shepherd.

He told the board in 1954, "For some time, we have been in touch with the Mennonite Central Committee with regard to setting up a program called the Volunteer Service of the Mennonite Church.

"As you know, the Mennonites are conscientious objectors and when a boy arrives at draft age, instead of serving in the Armed Forces he is allowed to work

191

for two years in an institution approved by the U.S. Army. The men are under what is known as the IW Program and the women under the Volunteer Service program of the Mennonite Church.

"We mentioned this about a year ago. The unit was to come the first of September, and then it was put off five or six times. They arrived March 22, three from Minnesota, one from Kansas and one from Illinois. We are well pleased with their services.

"Some time ago, I spoke of the importance of procuring the proper individuals for our staff. If we hired three or four people who were crude, rough and undisciplined, it would not be long before one could change the entire complexion of The Good Shepherd Home.

"These five Mennonites exert a powerful influence for good. They take a wholesome and active interest in The Good Shepherd Home.

"The Central Committee receives seventy-five dollars per month for each one, but this is not paid to them individually. It is sent directly to the Mennonite Central Committee at Akron, Pennsylvania. They, in turn, get ten dollars per month spending money.

"The men serve two years, the time required of them by the government, and the women volunteer to give a year.

"They could work elsewhere at a recognized institution and receive a full salary. But these five are giving freely of themselves in a gesture of Christian service."

There would be more than fifty Mennonites who would serve Good Shepherd in the ensuing years.

* * *

Connie Raker saw Good Shepherd as a Protestant Boys Town. It had come to be known as "the Home with a heart." It attracted the love and support of many Catholics, Jews and those of other Protestant denominations beyond its Lutheran origins and continued ties.

And that led Connie into some battles with the

192

hierarchy of his church over schemes that eventually would have the effect of confining Good Shepherd's fund-raising efforts to Lutherans. He wouldn't be Papa Raker's son if he had gone through life without some fights with church officialdom.

Connie had repelled a proposal at synod in the early 1960s, by a narrow margin, that would have called for establishing a Lutheran United Way for the social agencies on synod's territory. It was asking Good Shepherd to give up its mailing lists and its right to solicit alone in its own behalf.

Then came a proposal by the leadership of the entire denomination that church-related agencies like Good Shepherd have their entire board elected by the church, rather than the two-thirds synod elected to Good Shepherd.

At one point in 1966 in his frustration, Connie told the board, "There have been times I actually disliked the word Lutheran."

He regretted the statement almost as soon as he gave it. Longtime friend and board member M. Luther Wahrmann took him to task for it. And at the very next meeting, Connie admitted that Wahrmann was right, that he had been too harsh.

"It's not the church that I have any objections to. It's a combination of the organization within the church and the term 'Lutheran' which isolates us from the life of other Christians.

"We are here to serve because we are Christians. We will serve those in need whether Christian or not.

"Some people think we are supported by the Lutheran Church. We are not—in an organized way. We don't get anything from synod or the Lutheran Church. But we do receive help from individual Christians and even from various congregations of those two bodies."

He was much more eloquent in the earlier battle over synod's federated appeal idea.

No other institution in the United Lutheran Church crosses not only synodical borders but denominational borders as we do, Connie proclaimed to the Good Shepherd board.

"In all its years, The Good Shepherd Home has asked synod only the opportunity to present its cause. Given that opportunity, it was the burden of the Home to convince individuals of the merit of its work."

Good Shepherd always cared for the physically handicapped, children or adults, regardless of money, creed, color or nationality. And it continues to have under its roof those of many denominations and creeds.

Connie said this uniqueness to serve has brought a uniqueness in response. There'd be no way for Good Shepherd to go through its lists to determine which friends are Lutheran and which are not.

Another factor the church should consider is that Good Shepherd gets support from all over the country. "There's a marked parallel between The Good Shepherd Home of Allentown, Pennsylvania, and the Roman Catholic institution of Boys Town in Omaha," Connie said.

"All know that Boys Town receives much Protestant money. The Good Shepherd Home in turn receives much Roman Catholic help. And Jews have always been favorably disposed toward our work because of our desire to help regardless of race or creed."

Finally, a federated fund would hurt Good Shepherd the most when it came to estates.

People would include Good Shepherd in their wills, he said. "It is just beyond belief that people would remember in their will a vague impersonal federated fund."

Synod's federated fund idea died. So did the church's proposal to have all board members picked by synod. ❖

18: BOARD PRESIDENTS

It would not take many of the wrong kind of people to change the whole personality of The Good Shepherd Home.

Connie Raker
January 13, 1953

When Muhlenberg College got a new president in 1937, Papa Raker provided a typical Good Shepherd welcome with a picture and write-up in *Sweet Charity*. And also typical with him was to include a little history lesson and a touch of Raker prophesy.

The item on Dr. Levering Tyson read:

"Muhlenberg College was named after Henry Melchior Muhlenberg, the patriarch of the Lutheran Church in America. In the seventy years of history, the college has had four presidents: The Rev. Dr. Frederick A. Muhlenberg (ten years), the Rev. Dr. Benjamin Sadler (nine years), the Rev. Dr. Theodore L. Seip (eighteen years) and the Rev. Dr. John A.W. Haas (thirty-two years). All these presidents were ministers of the Gospel.

"The fifth president, Levering Tyson, A.B., A.M., Litt.D., was elected president by the college board of trustees at the semiannual meeting January 19, 1937. Dr. Tyson is the first layman elected president of the college and will assume the duties of the office July 1.

"Fifty years ago, the Church would not have elected a layman as president. Things are changing. Men and ideas are changing. The laymen of the Lutheran Church have become so helpful and influential in all branches of church work that when Dr. Tyson was elected president, it was with the hearty approval of the Church and the friends of the institution.

"The women of the Lutheran Church are doing such noble work in all branches of church work that in years to come Muhlenberg College may even elect a woman as president."

Yes, Papa, and so may The Good Shepherd Home.

Over its eighty years, the Home has been guided by ninety-seven trustees, Papa and Connie Raker and eighty-seven other men, Mama Raker and seven other women—three of those women sitting on the board in this eightieth anniversary year.

The board began in 1909 with five self-appointed members, including Mama and Papa Raker. Five was the legal minimum. And actually, it was the Rakers who enlisted the entire board.

The conditions they set said at least four had to be members of the Evangelical Lutheran Church and at least three, members of Ministerium congregations.

With increasing pressure from critics within the Ministerium over the next decade, the board agreed to increase its size to seven—but the increase would be of people it picked. For several years around the end of World War I, there were six.

Then, in 1921, it acquiesced in letting the Ministerium choose that seventh member. It unanimously elected the Rev. Dr. Solomon E. Ochsenford of Bath at its convention that year and he took his seat on the board immediately after.

Around 1930, the board was expanded to eleven with two of the eleven being elected by the Ministerium.

In the 1941 issue of *Sweet Charity* that carried Papa's death, the list of trustees for the first time showed four chosen by synod. This was carrying out a new bylaw provision which read:

"The Home shall be under the management of a board of trustees consisting of not less than ten nor more than fifteen trustees, four of whom shall be members of and elected by the Ministerium . . . and the others by the board itself. Of these trustees, two may be women. No salaried officer or employee of the Home excepting the superintendent shall be eligible to election as a trustee."

There was only one woman on the board at that time, Edna Hart, the longtime president of the Woman's Auxiliary. And over the board's seventy-nine years of existence, it was an all-male body forty-four of those years. It would not be until 1981 that the board would have two women members, Midge Mosser and Pauline MacDonald Ruloff.

In 1949, Muhlenberg College sociologist Morris Greth used Good Shepherd as his first subject in a study of the inner mission institutions within the territory of the Ministerium and their ties to synod.

Perhaps prompted by that, Connie cautioned the board:

"There have been many institutions in our country founded by church denominations which have long since dissociated themselves from the church which founded them. While there is no chance of this happening at present, who can say what might happen years from now," he reported in April 1949.

"I think it would be well if we studied a possible change which would make the tie between The Good Shepherd Home and the Ministerium closer. At least, there should be something in the charter or bylaws which would prevent the Home from ever being shaken from its moorings."

The board referred the matter to its executive committee.

Connie was back before the board with the same concerns a year later, citing Lankenau Hospital's being lost to the Lutheran Church.

"It would be best if we united ourselves even closer to the Church. This could be done by increasing the number of members elected by the Ministerium. Our board membership is fifteen. We would like to recommend that eight, a majority, be elected by the Ministerium."

The board took no action.

Finally in 1955, the board saw it Connie's way by revising the bylaws, calling for fifteen trustees plus the superintendent. Nine had to be members of and chosen by synod.

The revision also simply eliminated the prior line that seemed to limit the number of women to two.

That has undergone further revision since. Now, in this eightieth anniversary year, the bylaws call for nineteen trustees, two-thirds of them chosen by the executive board of the Northeastern Pennsylvania Lutheran Synod—a segment of the old Ministerium whose territory includes Allentown.

The remaining trustees have to include an active member of the Good Shepherd Rehabilitation Hospital staff.

Over these nearly eighty years, that board has been presided over by eight men—Papa Raker and three other Lutheran ministers and four active Lutheran laymen: a meat plant owner, a judge, a paint company proprietor and the operator of a food processing business.

The title was president of the board until 1983 when it became "chairman." Those board leaders have been:

Rev. Dr. John H. Raker	1909 - 1916
Wilson Arbogast	1916 - 1924
Rev. Dr. George Gebert	1924 - 1936
Rev. Dr. Conrad Wilker	1936 - 1944
Judge James F. Henninger	1944 - 1959
Rev. Dr. Henry J. Pflum	1959 - 1962
Tilghman G. Fenstermaker	1962 - 1974
Julian W. Newhart	1974 -

This book has more than introduced Papa Raker. And it has touched a bit upon Wilson Arbogast's leadership in the $100,000 campaign of 1916. Even before that, Arbogast saw to it that his meat packing plant was donating about $500 worth of meats to the Home each year.

He was hampered by illness much of the time he was board president. At his death, *Sweet Charity* called him one of the Home's best friends.

The psalmist says, "Blessed is the man in whose

spirit there is no guile." Papa often thought of Arbogast in connection with the beautiful expression of Jesus when he spoke of Nathaniel: "Behold, an Israelite without guile."

* * *

Dr. Gebert served the entire forty-seven years of his ministry at Zion Lutheran Church in Tamaqua. A massive stone church was built during his ministry. When he died in 1940 at age eighty-two, he was the oldest minister in the Ministerium of Pennsylvania.

Papa first met George Gebert when they were students at Muhlenberg. Papa said in a eulogy, "If it had not been for Dr. Gebert, I would have packed my things and gone home. I had such implicit confidence in him then that I was willing to lay my immortal soul into his hands. I realized he had been with Jesus.

"In all these fifty-seven years since, I have had no occasion to change my mind.

"I do not know what we could have done at the Home if it had not been for Dr. Gebert's help and influence. Many of the advanced ideas at the Home came from his fertile mind and heart.

"Before putting up the boys' dormitory costing over $100,000 for sixty crippled orphan boys and the old people's building costing over $100,000 years ago, a committee of the Home visited institutions for days and days.

"Dr. Gebert was always in the rear, and we thought he was a little slow. When we came back, we found out, however, that he had a lot we did not have."

State inspectors hailed the boys' dorm with its ramps and elevators as the most convenient building for disabled people in the country. A woman from the federal government who toured the old people's quarters said this was the first home in 150 she had visited with private lavatories in each private room.

"The credit for most of these up-to-date conveniences belonged to Dr. Gebert," Papa said.

"We did not wait for the funeral to say this, but said it a number of times to friends in his presence—'in honor preferring one another.' He ignored it, but knew it was the truth."

*   *   *

Dr. Conrad Wilker was pastor of St. Michael's Lutheran in Allentown from 1926 until his death in 1944. But it was his prior service at two congregations in Philadelphia that instilled in him a love for inner mission work. Next to his parish, inner mission work took a goodly share of his life. He had a rule to make at least three pastoral calls a day.

He came to St. Michael's in downtown Allentown despite warnings from friends that the community was changing, populations were shifting and a popular minister had just left. Expect a loss in membership, they said.

He came, he worked and St. Michael's—the church of Aunt Mary Eisenhard—thrived. It grew by 900 members during his tenure. He involved himself with Allentown Hospital and social agencies in the community.

And during his unexpectedly brief years as president of the Good Shepherd board, the Home renovated its former Red Cross building to house twenty of its workers, a new wing was built on the old folks building and many internal improvements were accomplished.

*   *   *

Judge James F. Henninger was once introduced at a Lutheran Church convention with a flourish by Dr. Franklin Clark Fry as James Flynn Henninger.

Quipped the judge in response, "That middle name is just a little mustard on a crock of sauerkraut."

Or as Connie Raker explained in giving his eulogy at the judge's funeral in 1970, "One of his grandparents was Irish, so he called himself an Irish octoroon. In this chaotic world, we can use more men of granite with a Bible in one hand and a bit of Irish laughter in their hearts."

Though a small man physically, Henninger was a

200

giant within what was then the United Lutheran Church in America—a member of its executive committee as well as a member of the executive board of the Ministerium and the Lutheran World Federation.

Connie said the mind of the nation was on other matters during the trying years of World War II. "To care for, educate and rehabilitate the handicapped remained the prime purpose of The Good Shepherd Home, but new problems were constantly added."

Adequate help was difficult to secure, especially trained help. Then, the government took 213 acres of Good Shepherd's farm for an airfield.

"From the standpoint of national defense, we realized this was necessary, but nonetheless it was difficult," Connie says.

"Here, the guiding genius of Judge Henninger made itself felt. He gave the board and the entire Good Shepherd Home family a sense of well-being and solidity.

"The knowledge we had a man of such stature overseeing our enterprise was one that inspired confidence. In spite of all the turmoil of the period, our morale was high and it was primarily due to him."

In an anniversary address the judge gave in 1943, he said, "It becomes important to bring home the strange fact that the greater the prosperity of the Home, the greater is its financial burden. While this Home may prosper, it can never grow rich. The more prosperous we become, the greater our responsibilities and the greater our need of your help.

"Some years ago, there came to our notice a crippled boy, then an inmate in a Florida almshouse. He had absolutely no claim upon our charity, excepting his dire need and our ability to help.

"We gladdened many years of his life to our credit. But he, by his gracious disposition, developed in our atmosphere of love and understanding, more than repaid all our effort by emanating good cheer wherever he was.

"When he passed away a short time ago, our loss was the greater because we remembered our hesitation in accepting our responsibility to him.

"Will you, who both know and understand what we aim to do and could do if only given the means, become our evangels to spread the Gospel of the Good Shepherd as it is exemplified and brought to fruition in this, The Good Shepherd Home?"

* * *

Dr. Pflum served the pulpit of Christ Lutheran Church in Allentown from 1943 to 1961. His interest in Good Shepherd was aroused soon after his call to that church.

Sweet Charity said, "He felt that this Home for crippled children and old folks, regardless of faith, creed or religion, was performing a vitally important work that would have to be expanded as the years went by.

"Consequently, he welcomed election to the Home's board of trustees and served in any capacity in which he could be helpful. His interest and devotion were not unnoticed by his fellow trustees. The result was his election as president of the board at its annual meeting in 1959."

When he decided to retire from the ministry in 1961 because of his advancing years and his health, he said, "My heart is still here in my congregation and at The Good Shepherd Home."

* * *

Tilghman G. "Til" Fenstermaker of Emmaus, president of Allentown Paint Manufacturing Co., headed the board for a dozen years in an era of expansion and growth. His congregation was Faith Lutheran in Whitehall, where he was treasurer for twenty-five years.

Family involvement with Good Shepherd had been a longtime thing. His father, Henry E. Fenstermaker, led one of the campaign teams in the $100,000 drive of 1916.

The summer of 1965 saw the dedication of the $830,000 Good Shepherd Rehabilitation Center. A twenty-two-bed Rehabilitation Hospital wing costing

$410,000 was opened in October 1967. And shortly thereafter the Home signed an agreement with Blue Cross to cover costs of patients' rehabilitation services at the hospital. Medicare approval also was granted.

The year 1972 brought the dedication of a $250,000 addition to the Good Shepherd Workshop that doubled the floor space and placed the entire vocational rehabilitation program in one building.

Connie characterized Til as "optimistic and forward-thinking, a jovial good-natured man with a wealth of stories for every occasion. His sense of loyalty went deeper than most people can imagine. I believe his love for his church and Good Shepherd ranked with his love for his wife and family."

*   *   *

Julian W. Newhart of Coplay is still making his mark as the head of the board in this eightieth anniversary year. The title was changed to chairman in 1983.

He has been the board leader through the changing of administrators from Connie Raker to Dale Sandstrom. He directed the board when it authorized construction of the Conrad W. Raker Center for the profoundly disabled and the massive expansions in the rehabilitation facilities from one end to the other of the 500 block of St. John Street. And he was a leader in seeing that the name was the Conrad W. Raker Center.

Dale Sandstrom describes Newhart as someone with visionary thinking—but with his feet on the ground. "He's in the conservative mode. Yet he'll move out in a venturesome way, especially for Good Shepherd.

"He's seen people come to the hospital and what it's done for their lives. He's deep into rehabilitation. He can also take a look at a balance sheet and ask some pretty penetrating questions."

Newhart's record at Good Shepherd goes on. . . .

*   *   *

Connie Raker once told the board, "It is impossible to overestimate the beneficial work done for The Good Shepherd Home by these women of the Ladies' Auxiliary."

They have contributed hundreds of thousands of dollars to various building projects and sponsored events that have raised tens of thousands more. They have used their skills in a multitude of ways to make clothing and other articles that have transformed Good Shepherd into a place just a bit homier for its residents than it would have without their touch.

They involved themselves in the actual care of the guests, something Connie called a work of serving love. For instance, they made sure the young girls had new outfits for confirmation.

Bazaars, fairs and dinners were the original methods of fund-raising. Later, these were augmented by antique shows, hobby shows, teas, fashion and flower shows, plays in which members of the auxiliary participated and art exhibits.

Just since 1952, records compiled by Emily Evans show the auxiliary treasury provided more than $100,000 to various Good Shepherd projects and, atop that, pledged $50,000 toward the 1988 hospital expansion.

Sometimes, auxiliary gifts were modest amounts that spoke of personal care and concern—a dollar or two to each of the guests for their birthdays, postage and cards for the guests, hymnals, a clock to Mama Raker as a birthday present or an English New Testament for Connie Raker on the twenty-fifth anniversary of his ordination into the Lutheran ministry.

Other times, these were gifts in the thousands of dollars for carpeting, shades for the auditorium, furniture, a new organ or for the building fund. One of those larger donations was in honor of Connie Raker with the opening of Raker Center.

In 1953, during the tenure of Arline Trexler as president, each of the nearly 700 members was given a dollar for six months to increase by using their talents. They returned with $5,500.

At the time he became superintendent, Connie declared, "Women form the backbone of the modern church. Women are the task force of many agencies for the betterment of society. So it is at The Good

Shepherd Home.

"The Ladies' Auxiliary has been of far more value to The Good Shepherd Home in its program of helping the most helpless who have none to help them than can ever be added up in dollars and cents."

His father phrased it another way in a single paragraph in a 1931 *Sweet Charity*: "The consecrated women of the Lutheran Church are beginning to do in the church what they always did in The Good Shepherd Home, that is, assert themselves."

The founding organization was the Allentown Auxiliary on August 26, 1909. As *The Morning Call* reported: "Some time ago, an enthusiastic orphans' home man of Allentown said, 'Get your ladies organized for The Good Shepherd Home, and you will have the best helpers any institution of mercy can secure.'

"Believing this to be true, an invitation was extended to the ladies of Allentown who are interested in this institution of mercy for crippled orphans, infant orphans and old people to meet at the Home on Thursday afternoon, August 26. The object was to organize for effective work at the Home."

Papa Raker opened the session with prayer and then outlined "the great work that the Home is expected to accomplish." Mama was elected temporary president while the group chose these founding officers:

Miss Laura V. Keck of St. John's Lutheran, president; Mrs. Sula Stetler of St. Stephen's, first vice president; Miss Carrie Bauer of St. Luke's, second vice president; Mrs. Otto Meyer of St. Peter's (Ridge Avenue), third vice president; Mrs. Edward Deily of Grace, fourth vice president; Mrs. Frank Lehman of St. Joseph's, fifth vice president; Mrs. Robert W. Kurtz of St. Michael's, secretary, and Mrs. R.S. Diehl of Christ, treasurer.

That array of leadership touched about every Lutheran church in town.

It was under Keck's tenure that the auxiliary contributed $5,000 toward the Home's $100,000 campaign of 1916. Several campaign teams were also headed by women in that drive.

Keck was already a community leader before she ever got to the Good Shepherd Auxiliary.

She had charge of the YWCA in Allentown from 1899, just a year after its founding, until 1918. She worked in other capacities with the YWCA up to her death in 1928.

She was a charter member of the Missionary Society of the Allentown Lutheran Conference, organized in 1888. She was president 1897-1904 and again 1909-1912.

Obviously, she was right there at the founding of the Missionary Society along with Aunt Mary Eisenhard—going in the face of a clerical hierarchy who said there was no precedent for establishing a Missionary Society and who offered no encouragement.

Keck was also a charter member of the Woman's Club of Allentown and the senior auxiliary of Allentown Hospital.

She was among those in the county who spearheaded an unsuccessful drive in 1915 for a suffrage amendment to the Pennsylvania Constitution.

At her death, the *Chronicle & News* carried a picture of her at a railroad station, the caption noting she was Travelers' Aid secretary of Allentown. It added:

"Her kind interest, heart-felt concern and sympathetic aid was a blessing to hundreds of men, women and children from foreign countries who were assisted to friends and relatives in and about Allentown, and to many more who were directed on their rightful course of travel after stopping off at Allentown to change trains.

"For many years, Miss Keck was prominent in the work of Lutheran missions."

With the establishment of the Good Shepherd Auxiliary in Allentown, other units were formed in various communities shortly afterward, some appearing briefly, others lasting for years— Bethlehem, Birdsboro, Coopersburg, Friedensville, Harrisburg, Hegins, Jim Thorpe, Quakertown, Saucon Valley, South Bethlehem, Reading and Sellersville.

The founding unit in Allentown, however, has always been looked upon as the auxiliary with regular meetings across the years. Others were really satellite groups that tried to collect money each year for the Home.

For instance, Alice V. Kern in Coopersburg in those early days went to friends and neighbors—mostly women, but men too— in that community and nearby villages to get a dollar each year for Good Shepherd. And it was no coincidence that mechanics in that same Kern family donated their services in reconditioning the first used car Papa ever got.

When the Home supplied canning jars by the hundreds to be filled with any bounty of the fall harvest, the distribution and collection network was there with these auxiliary units. The canned foodstuffs helped Good Shepherd make it over those first winters, just as surely as did the coal supplied by the men of the Centurion Band of the Wilkes-Barre Conference.

Sweet Charity shows that perhaps a half dozen of the satellite auxiliaries existed through the 1950s. Then, they dropped off to just Allentown and Bethlehem. After 1975, it was one unit as it is today.

The general pattern in the early years of this century was for married women to go by their husband's first name in any formal listing. Edna Hart headed the auxiliary for twenty years (1923-1943) and served on the Home's board for nearly as long (1930-1949). Yet she was always Mrs. J. Maurice Hart on the pages of *Sweet Charity*, including for her obituary.

In keeping with the spirit of the 1980s, here are the names of the women who led the auxiliary:

Laura V. Keck	1913 - 1919	
Maude M. Pretz	1919 - 1923	
Edna S. Hart	1923 - 1943	
Anna L. Diefenderfer	1944 - 1948	
Esther Beer	1949 - 1952	
Arline Trexler	1953	
Isolde Wood	1954	
Erma Everitt	1955	
Anna L. Diefenderfer		1956
Mildred Kirchman	1957 - 1961	
Althea Yeager	1962 - 1964	
Florence Harwick	1965 - 1967	

Ruth Diehl	1968 - 1970
Marion Schlack	1970 - 1972
Winifred Bausch	1972 - 1974
Carolyn Sue Bonser	1974 - 1976
Edna Rader	1976 - 1978
Florine Rohrbach	1978 - 1982
Dorothy Christman	1982 - 1987
Evelyn Allen	1987

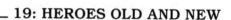

A crippled body is not an indication of a crippled mind.

Sweet Charity
May-June 1928

Connie Raker says he has lived among heroes at The Good Shepherd Home, and he has. But besides extolling those within the Home, the people of Good Shepherd have looked beyond its domain sometimes for heroes.

Papa and Mama Raker themselves, and Connie after them, have probably been considered heroes by many who have lived within the Home and perhaps even more by those from the outside.

One older Home boy, Russell Diefenderfer, said that in his view of who was the greatest woman in America, "Eleanor Roosevelt came in a close second to Mama."

And a fellow pastor told Papa, "God conferred a very great honor upon you, brother Raker, when he entrusted to you so faithful, so capable and so truly loyal a helpmeet in Mrs. Raker."

In a quiet way, Good Shepherd pointed to Helen Keller as a hero—using article after article by her in *Sweet Charity* in the early years on such topics as rehabilitation of the handicapped. Papa called this educated deaf and blind woman the marvel of the world. And he asked: "If Miss Keller's misfortunes were sent for a purpose, what of our slight afflictions at The Good Shepherd Home?"

Papa cited other heroes beyond the confines of Good Shepherd in a piece in the May-June 1928 *Sweet Charity*:

"One day while U.S. Customs officers were busily examining immigrants, they were confronted by a little chap so deformed he could hardly walk. They were on the verge of sending him back when some of the boy's relatives 'showed up' and promised to take care of him.

"This little boy was Charles Steinmetz (1865-1923), the greatest electrical wizard of the age. The man who produced thunder and lightning by the power of his will. The man whose scientific value to the world, next to Edison, cannot be measured in dollars and cents.

"When we see pictures of this man, we always see him leaning on his desk, working. He always said it was better and easier for him to work while in this position."

As a boy of ten, John Raker met another lad his age who loved to read. One day, this boy took him into an old attic where he kept his books. John saw a book there called *Treasure Island* by Robert Louis Stevenson. This book fascinated him. He picked it up. He was to read it through many times.

Later on, young John Raker read another book by the same author, *Dr. Jekyll and Mr. Hyde.*

And those two books created within him a desire to study the life of the author. Great was his surprise when he found that Robert Louis Stevenson was a man who could not move from his bed.

On the pages of *Sweet Charity*, Papa would point to these lessons from childhood.

"There were many men who were cripples and became great," his *Sweet Charity* writings said. "If we were to study the biographies of Alexander Pope, Byron, Milton and Heine, we would find that they were crippled. No! A crippled body is not an indication of a crippled mind. That is just an opinion which is formed by an employer."

He called the crippled child one who had borne the cross of centuries. That child needs help. "He must first of all be found, then have orthopedic aid, be educated and last of all employed."

Papa, of course, without using the word heroes, was citing those right there at Good Shepherd.

"We have a boy without arms," he reminded *Sweet Charity* readers in 1928 of Raymond Myers. "He had been taught to do many things with his toes. When this boy was in junior high, the teacher, after careful study of the boy, found that he loved to paint pictures. She got the students to gather a little money and purchase art lessons for him.

"It is the duty of education to find the talents of the pupil and develop them. Our whole education system has utterly failed if it does not find the talents of the child."

The Rakers were unreconstructed Democrats, *Sweet Charity* even quoting the guest speaker at the 1936 Raker family reunion telling the gathering that his research of the family revealed "that there had always been too many Democrats among the Rakers."

Papa was an avid fan of William Jennings Bryan. He had voted for Bryan for president three times and vehemently declared he would gladly do so again. But *Sweet Charity* was never turned into a partisan publication. The closest it got was this exchange in Pregnant Thoughts in the September-October 1932 issue:

One of the boys at The Good Shepherd Home said: "Papa Raker, I believe you are going to vote for Roosevelt because he is a cripple."

Papa's answer: "That may have something to do with it, and you as a cripple should consider it as a compliment."

Through those Depression years, there were perhaps a phrase here and a line there that indicated the crippled of Good Shepherd were well aware that a man crippled with polio, Franklin Roosevelt, was president of the United States—sort of "one of us" has made it.

It would be a generation later—starting in 1976— that The Good Shepherd Home of Allentown, Pennsylvania, would reach across this nation to honor individuals with various disabilities who have made outstanding achievements in life.

It would be called the Handicapped Hall of Fame.

It would be the idea of Ray Crissey, director of The Good Shepherd Rehabilitation Hospital.

By the eightieth anniversary year, Good Shepherd had honored fourteen individuals with its Handicapped Hall of Fame award. They would include people high in the federal government. They would also include two Home boys, Carl Odhner and Jeff Steinberg.

As Connie Raker explained at the first Handicapped Hall of Fame ceremony:

"Throughout its history, The Good Shepherd Home has seen the indomitable spirit, strength and faith that has permitted those with severe disabilities to overcome their many handicaps and go on to live useful, productive and even outstanding lives.

"This award is made in tribute to that spirit."

The recipients:

1976 U.S. Sen. Daniel Inouye
     Hawaii

1977 Max Cleland
     Director of U.S. Veterans Administration

1978 Roy Campanella
     Former Dodger catcher

1979 Carl F. Odhner
     GSH Vice President

1980 Dr. Henry Viscardi Jr.
     President, Human Resources Center Abilities

1981 Judge Leonard Staisey
     Allegheny County Court

1982 Rev. Harold Wilke
     Director, Healing Community

1983 U.S. Sen. Robert Dole
     Kansas

1984 James S. Brady
     White House Press Secretary

1985 Dr. Anne Carlsen
     Anne Carlsen School

1986 Edward M. Kennedy Jr
       Facing the Challenge

     Mary Nemec Doremus
       National Challenge Committee on Disability

1987 Jeff Steinberg
       Singer, Motivator

     Justin W. Dart Jr.
       Commissioner, Rehabilitation Services
       Administration

Judge Staisey is blind. The others make up quite a collection of wheelchairs and artificial limbs.

They also make up a tremendous mountain of human achievement.

Crissey, the director of the rehabilitation hospital, says he had talked to Dr. Raker about establishing an award in honor of his father, to call it the John H. Raker Rehabilitation Excellence Award.

"We talked about it several times," Crissey says. "He didn't go with that at the moment. So I said if you're not ready to do that, let's establish an award to honor the handicapped. It was to honor those who have made a major contribution to the field of rehabilitation and at the same time have some handicap of their own to overcome."

Crissey heads the selection committee. And prior recipients are sort of honorary members of that committee. Some of them have offered suggestions.

In presenting the first award to Senator Inouye in 1976, Connie Raker said, "A good deal of prayer and thought preceded our decision to establish this award.

"We are giving it to one who has demonstrated the belief so strongly adhered to by The Good Shepherd Home—that the existence of handicapped conditions, regardless of their severity, need not prevent a person and, indeed, may inspire a person to outstanding accomplishments for the good and benefit of their fellow men."

Inouye lost his right arm in the closing days of World War II. His hopes of becoming a surgeon shattered by his disability, he turned to studying

213

government and economics. He was elected Hawaii's first congressman in 1959. He was elected to the U.S. Senate in 1962 where he still serves as Good Shepherd reaches its eightieth year.

* * *

When Max Cleland, Good Shepherd's 1977 Hall of Famer, was sworn in as administrator of the U.S. Veterans Administration, President Jimmy Carter said of him, "He has overcome the handicap of disabilities suffered in war in a way that has never demanded sympathy. He never asks for special consideration."

At thirty-four, he was the youngest administrator of the VA and the first Vietnam veteran to head it. Cleland lost both legs and part of his right arm in a grenade explosion near Khe Sanh in 1968 when he was an Army combat officer.

At the Good Shepherd ceremony, Cleland turned the attention upon another person who had been injured by a grenade, Home boy Dino Katsiaris, an economist with the VA. "He's a shining light and an example to others," Cleland said of Dino.

Cleland told the gathering, "Hemingway said life breaks us all, but afterward many are stronger in the broken places. And I think that's the kind of life we would all like to live—to be stronger in the broken places."

* * *

Roy Campanella in 1978 was the first baseball Hall of Famer to become a member of the Handicapped Hall of Fame. A catching great with the Brooklyn Dodgers (1948-57) and one of the first black superstars in big league baseball, he was left almost completely paralyzed from injuries from a traffic accident in early 1958.

Sweet Charity said, "Over the years, his indomitable spirit and courage have enabled Campy to become an example to those whose handicaps are far less severe." He became a public relations man for the New York Mets, a sportscaster and a lecturer.

Campy told the Good Shepherd crowd, "With your help and time, you'd be surprised what you can do."

* * *

The September-October 1979 cover of *Sweet Charity* said it all about the presentation to Home boy Carl Odhner as that year's recipient. It was a picture of Carl being embraced by Connie Raker—two men whose lives had been so intertwined with Good Shepherd for more than a generation.

Connie called him "a man with a sense of purpose, but also a sense of humor, a handicapped person who never accepted that fact. He goes full tilt at anything he does."

And Carl said what a joy it is to be able to work in a profession such as rehabilitation where the basic principles are preserving and restoring human usefulness. "Good Shepherd is as much a spirit as it is a practice."

* * *

Dr. Henry Viscardi Jr., a man born with stumps for legs, was the 1980 recipient in a ceremony that included the dedication of the $5 million Conrad W. Raker Center.

In 1952, Viscardi gave up a personnel job in a textile mill, borrowed $8,000 and, in a vacant garage on Long Island, started a Human Resources Center to prove that the physically handicapped, if given the chance, can work efficiently in industry.

It gained international recognition. And for Good Shepherd, the work of Viscardi had a special meaning. In the mid-1950s, Connie Raker heard Viscardi speak at a Rotary meeting in New York City. "His inspiring words remained with me. With the help of the local business community, we opened our own Good Shepherd Workshop here on South Fifth Street in 1958," Connie recalled.

"It takes guts to be free," Viscardi told the

dedication audience. "The waste of life lies in love not given, talents not used."

* * *

Allegheny County Judge Leonard C. Staisey, who is blind, reminded the 1981 Good Shepherd Day audience that "the great handicap of the handicapped is not their handicap, but the attitude the public has toward them."

As a state senator in the early 1960s, he sponsored bills related to architectural barriers, child abuse, funding the Carnegie Institute Braille Library, and mental health and retardation.

As a county commissioner, he was instrumental in implementing affirmative action for the handicapped, county jobs for disabled Vietnam veterans and the building of three community college campuses with emphasis on access for the handicapped.

The ceremony for Staisey's elevation to the Handicapped Hall of Fame also included special recognition to blind Justin McDevitt of Rosemont and Charles O'Brien of Carlisle, a man who lost a leg in Vietnam. They were among nine disabled people who climbed 14,410-foot Mount Rainier that summer to observe the International Year of the Disabled Person.

* * *

The Rev. Dr. Harold Wilke, a man born without arms who developed an entire ministry for the handicapped, was added to the Handicapped Hall of Fame in 1982. He is a United Church of Christ minister and executive director of The Healing Community of White Plains, New York.

He developed total independence, maintaining, "That part is easy. The real challenge is learning to live securely and helpfully and leading others to lives of strength and creative happiness."

He lauded Good Shepherd: "You here recognize the enormous benefits, abilities and strengths that persons with disabilities have and the way they, therefore, teach the rest of us."

216

Special recognition awards went to Jim Coyne of Allentown and Diane Shemenski, a senior at Central Bucks, for courage in spite of their disabilities. Both are amputees who became champion handicapped skiers.

* * *

Kansas Sen. Robert J. Dole had the unusual distinction of being the only recipient of the Handicapped Hall of Fame award who did not attend the ceremony where it was presented. Instead, Dole was shown through a film made in Washington, D.C., for the 1983 awards program.

During World War II, Dole was twice wounded and twice decorated for heroism. He spent thirty-nine months in a hospital after being hit by machine gun fire in the Po Valley in Italy.

He was elected to the U.S. House of Representatives in 1960 and the U.S. Senate in 1968.

Three Good Shepherd alumni were also honored at that ceremony—Veterans Administration economist Dino Katsiaras, inspirational singer and motivator Jeff Steinberg and Douglas Kern, an engineer and businessman who was at Good Shepherd while a high school student because of a spinal cord injury from playing football.

Dale Sandstrom would later present Dole with his award in Washington.

* * *

"I'm thrilled to be honored by the premier rehabilitation institute in the nation," said White House press secretary James S. Brady, the 1984 inductee into the Handicapped Hall of Fame.

Brady was wounded in the head during a 1981 assassination attempt on President Reagan. He was honored as one who has "overcome a handicap and risen to a level of achievement that works for the good and benefit of others."

Good Shepherd honored him for his courage, his persistence and his physical embodiment of hope for the severely injured or handicapped.

Three local people were cited for honors at the ceremony: Kenneth "Wheels" McHenry, a paraplegic who was a Good Shepherd resident and wheelchair athlete during 1949-59; James W. Snyder Jr., who lost both legs in the Korean War, whose business and public career included being Good Shepherd controller 1961-73, and Geraldine "Granny" Yocum, who traveled in her power wheelchair from Bethlehem to Disney World in Florida.

What a touching footnote that Jim Brady's mother, Dorothy Brady, wrote later from her home in Centralia, Illinois.

"The Good Shepherd event was truly an inspiration to all of us. We came home with great satisfaction regarding the 'caring' shown to residents of Good Shepherd Home. I am going to speak to a church group using much of the material regarding Good Shepherd."

She noted that papers across the country had carried stories about her son getting the Good Shepherd award. And she closed with a thank you for giving Jim a ride back home to Arlington in a Good Shepherd van. "It was more comfortable than the car."

*   *   *

"To be truly handicapped is to be without feeling. You don't have that here," said Dr. Anne Carlsen, the 1985 Handicap Hall of Famer.

She was administrator emeritus of the Anne Carlsen School for the Physically Handicapped in Jamestown, North Dakota.

She was born with only stumps for arms, six inches of thigh for one leg and a twisted stump for the other. Despite lengthy stays in the hospital, she went on to acquire a Ph.D. and taught handicapped children for forty-seven years.

Others honored at the 1985 ceremony were all in wheelchairs: Attorney Doug Heir of Cherry Hill, New Jersey, world champion in the javelin at the 1984 World Wheelchair Games; Corrine Rotondo, former Good Shepherd patient with back injuries, a receptionist at Mack Trucks World Headquarters, and Mike King, who wheeled his way from Fairbanks, Alaska, to Washington, D.C.

* * *

Two things were decidedly different about the 1986 Hall of Fame program.

For the first time, two awards were given—to Mary Nemec Doremus, president of the National Challenge Committee on Disability with headquarters in Washington, D.C., and Edward M. Kennedy Jr., executive director of Facing the Challenge, with offices in Boston.

Second, two persons were cited posthumously for their outstanding contributions to the community— former Good Shepherd boy Ray Myers, the first armless person to get a driver's license in Pennsylvania, and Bonnie Gellman Simon, former director of the Philadelphia Mayor's Commission on People with Disabilities.

There was also an award to Ernie Stiegler, chairman of his own Allentown advertising agency.

* * *

A young man who provided some of the singing for years at Anniversary Day programs was inducted into the Handicapped Hall of Fame in 1987—Jeff Steinberg, inspirational singer, author, motivator and former Good Shepherd resident—and Justin W. Dart Jr., Commissioner of Rehabilitation for the U.S. Department of Education.

Steinberg was co-author of a recent book on his life story, *Masterpiece in Progress.* He was born without arms and with deformed legs. From a Jewish family and bar mitzvahed while at Good Shepherd, he became a born again Christian when he grew up. When he married, Jerry Falwell performed the ceremony.

His book at times seethed with bitterness that his parents had turned their backs on him in childhood with his multiple afflictions.

But it was an obviously softened Jeff Steinberg who addressed the Good Shepherd audience. Perhaps with writing the book he had purged the hurt and anger inside.

No honor was greater than from those he grew up with, he said. He asked: "How do you say thank you for love?" It was a special night, too, because his mother was there and heard him sing live for the first time. "I love you, Mom," Jeff called out from the stage.

Justin Dart from his wheelchair said, "Two hundred years is long enough for people with disabilities to wait to be first-class citizens. Now is the time to establish full equality."

There were also honors to four others for their achievements —Norma Jean Bancroft, a Good Shepherd resident who is among the top ten cerebral palsy athletes in the country; Dave Fowler, a Vietnam veteran who teaches skiing to amputees in the Poconos; Charles Gerras, a quadriplegic who is senior editor at Rodale Books in Emmaus, and Jim McGowan of Fort Washington, a paraplegic who left his wheelchair earlier that summer to try to swim the English Channel.

As an old *Sweet Charity* line so appropriately asks: "Where is your place in the sun?" ❖

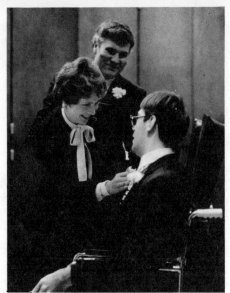

Dale and Lillian Sandstrom congratulate Tom Nestor upon being elected to the King's Court at the residents' annual ball, 1985.

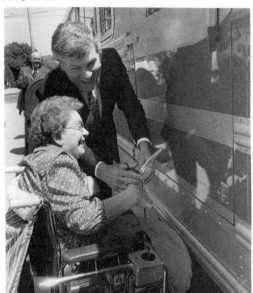

Good Shepherd president Dale E. Sandstrom helps Anna Mary Musser cut the ribbon for a new bus donated by the friends of Good Shepherd, 1986. In the background is Julian W. Newhart, chairman of the board of trustees.

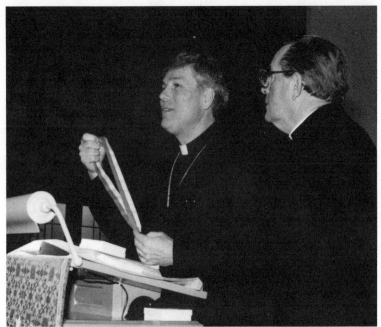

Dale Sandstrom presents Connie Raker with the first John H. and D. Estella Raker Memorial Award in recognition of his lifelong service to people with disabilities, 1986. The ceremony took place in Papa Raker's church, Grace Evangelical Lutheran Church in Allentown.

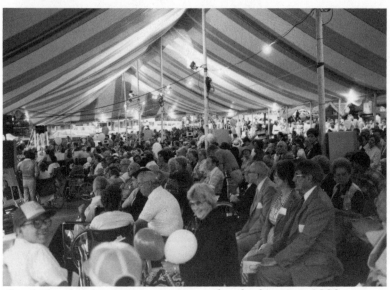

Good Shepherd Day ceremonies under the big tent, 1986.

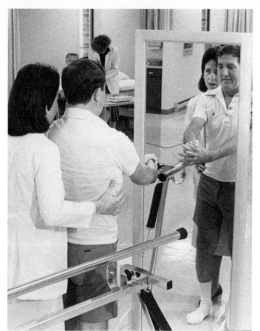

Physical therapist and outpatient center director Maggie McMenamin gives Larry Shafer a steadying hand at Good Shepherd Outpatient Services/Cedar Crest, 1986.

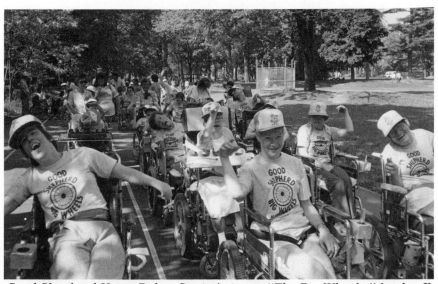

Good Shepherd Home Raker Center's team, "The Big Wheels," leads off the parade at the United Cerebral Palsy Association games in Philadelphia, 1986.

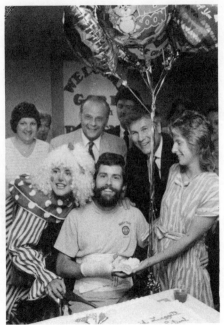

Good Shepherd Rehabilitation Hospital welcomes its 15,000th patient, 1986. Front row: clown Karen Mattos, David Leggett, Jenny Miller. Back row: Linda Hetherington, Joie Barry, Lehigh County executive David Bausch, Joseph O'Donnell and Dale Sandstrom. Photo courtesy of Naomi Halperin, Morning Call.

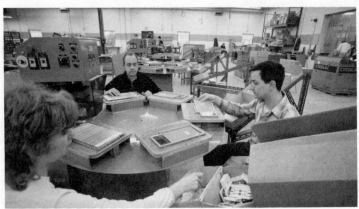

Donna Kemmerer, William Covely and Jeff Kratzer assemble toys at Good Shepherd Industrial Services, 1986.

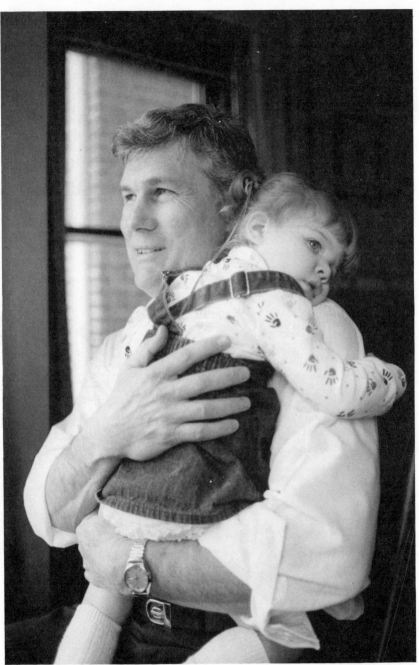

Dale Sandstrom and little Erin Santa at Good Shepherd's Early Childhood Center, 1987.

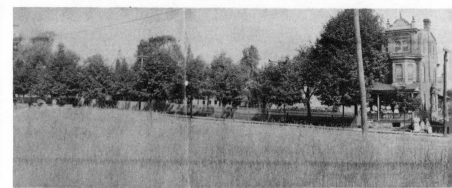

St. John Street, 1908.

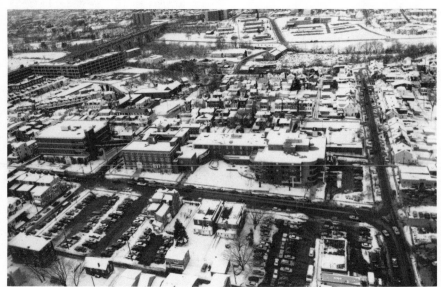

St. John Street, 1988.

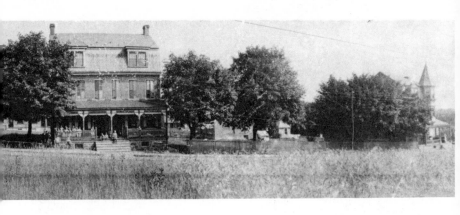

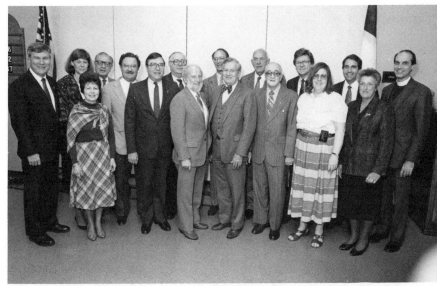

The Good Shepherd board of trustees, 1988: The Rev. Dale Sandstrom; Kris L. Shafer; Midge Mosser; Harold E. Everett, M.D.; John Raker Hudders, Esq.; David D. Hoffman; Julian W. Newhart; the Rev. Richard C. Wolf; Charles L. Knecht, M.D.; George S. Boyer, M.D.; Gil Castree; Robert D. Edwards; Raymond E. Holland; Tamar Earnest, M.D.; Robert W. Knipe; Evelyn Allen and the Rev. Dr. Gilbert B. Furst. Not shown are Jacob R. Esser; James W. Fisher Jr.; The Rev. Denton R. Kees; Edward J. Lentz, Esq.; Paul E. Lentz; Peter W. Likins, Ph.D.; John J. McGee; Walter J. Okunski, M.D.; The Hon. Donald L. Ritter; Richard M. Snyder and Ronald Young.

227

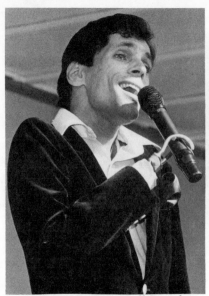

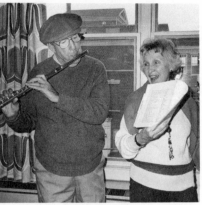

Connie and Grace Raker caroling at Good Shepherd Home Raker Center on Christmas morning, 1987.

Motivational singer Jeff Steinberg was inducted into the Handicapped Hall of Fame, 1987.

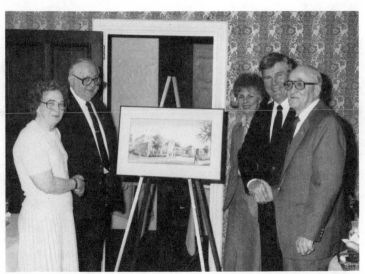

Julian Newhart, Institutional Advancement vice president Lona Farr and Dale Sandstrom congratulate Marian and Bob Edwards, at left and at right, at a 1987 celebration of their gift of $750,000 to Good Shepherd's endowment fund. Shown is a rendering of the Robert and Marian Edwards Center, named in honor of their gift, which now houses the Industrial Medicine and Vocational Services programs.

The world is a great big round ball with steps all over it like goose bumps.

Carl Odhner
Sweet Charity
January-February 1950

Papa Raker offered a rather prophetic "thought for future architects" in the January-February 1931 issue of *Sweet Charity*. It was tied to a bit of a parable involving Verna Hoppes, a disabled Home girl who would go on to college, marriage and an independent life.

Central Junior High principal Louis Dieruff had sent a letter praising Verna's work in her first year at the school. "Through preparation, careful faithful attention to duty and industry, she has won the commendation of her teachers," Dieruff wrote to Papa.

Dieruff's letter, of course, was reprinted in *Sweet Charity* along with Papa's comments on how delighted the Home was with her achievements.

"Verna is one of our cheerful, faithful and dependable girls," Papa said. When she came to the Home, she was too crippled to attend public school, church or Sunday school. She attended the special school at the Home.

"By constant physical efforts, she has improved wonderfully," *Sweet Charity* said. "There are some things the crippled must do for themselves in order to improve and succeed."

Papa recalled that one time, somewhat earlier, Verna was slowly walking with her crutches along the street with some other girls. He heard them talking about pictures. He suspected she had been to the moving picture show.

When the chance presented itself, he asked, "Verna, how is it you are too crippled to go to public school, church and Sunday school, but it seems you can go to the movies?"

Verna responded, "Papa, you know I would like to go to public school, church and Sunday school. But they have high steps.

"At the movies, they have no steps at all."

*   *   *

Carl Odhner has spent much of his adult life trying to knock down the physical barriers that face wheelchair people like himself. Sometimes he's resorted to humor to achieve his ends— willing to poke fun at himself as well as others. And he and his allies have had some rather sizable accomplishments.

He even took on Connie Raker indirectly once when Connie headed the Redevelopment Authority of Allentown, which had just completed the rebuilding of four blocks of Hamilton Street in downtown Allentown into what was rechristened the Hamilton Mall.

It was a mall that was not wheelchair accessible. The curbs prevented it from being so. And Odhner got the mayor and some other officials out on that mall in wheelchairs to demonstrate the problems—just before Governor Milton Shapp was supposed to come into town to bless all that a state grant hath wrought. The city quickly installed blacktop inclines at the curb at the end of each block.

In this eightieth anniversary year, Carl, vice president for human services, is a fixture in the Good Shepherd community.

Not bad for a kid who grew up in suburban Philadelphia with a silver spoon attached to his wheelchair. He was hit by polio at nine weeks. He was waited on. He didn't have to do a thing.

So it was a jolt when he arrived at The Good Shepherd Home in September 1942 and about the first thing they asked him to do was to help dry the dishes. He quickly found this was a place where everybody was asked to pitch in.

Carl arrived with the ultra-minimum of fanfare. There was simply the word "applications" and the name "Fritz Odhner" after it in Connie's report to the board on September 9, 1942.

Carl was introduced to *Sweet Charity* readers in the March-April 1943 issue, looking uncharacteristically somber from his wheelchair. "Fritz has a very full and beautiful voice, and we are arranging to have a voice teacher for him."

Sometimes in the evening a nurse at the piano would accompany Carl. Soon, others would be attracted and gather around to join in the singing.

In 1948, that baritone voice would win for the Home the first television set it had. Carl survived the early rounds of competition to be among the final twenty in a contest sponsored by the Allentown Musical Exchange and Dorney Park. He sang "Without a Song." He won.

As Home boy Morris Blinderman wrote in *Sweet Charity*, "It seemed unbelievable to his hazed and happy well-wishing crippled buddies at the Home. They had dreamed of having a television set—and now Carl had made their dream come really true."

In 1950, Carl at twenty-one had some rather prophetic words to share at a meeting with a group of normals, words that came to be shared with the wider audience of readers of *Sweet Charity*:

"These crippled limbs stand as a challenge. The fact that the limbs are impaired does not stop the soul from feeling that this world is too little for an ambitious nature.

"The worst handicap the physically disabled have is a misunderstood 'pity' and ignorance toward our disabilities.

"A normal person can never know the thrill a handicapped knows just from learning to lift yourself from a bed to a wheelchair.

"The simple everyday moves you make, without ever noticing how you do it, are made by the crippled with careful thought and planning. Some of the complicated pulls and twists we use may seem like a weary task, but really they are quite simple to use. We are proud of what we can do for ourselves."

Carl said there were difficulties some cripples can never hope to conquer—such as steps. "The greatest disability we face is steps—the kind you walk up and down.

"There is many a youngster who would not be sitting at home in a wheelchair or with crutches if his school was constructed with consideration that someday a crippled would attend.

"I have always thought that a bill should be passed by state or federal government whereby facilities for the handicapped be a requirement just as fire escapes and proper lighting. One consultation with a crippled person and the architect would know just what to do—draw in an elevator."

Carl had other suggestions—an entrance at ground level or with a ramp. "There are a thousand suggestions that could be made by crippled people . . ." And if you do these things for schools, do them for churches, too.

"One of the best I have ever heard is to have small ramps constructed of cement on the street corners. If such a plan were carried out, a third of those now on wheelchairs with no hope of ever leaving them could get jobs."

And young Carl maintained to the assembled normals that they needed help from the cripples just as much as the cripples did from them. They had to get to understand each other.

"As many of you know, I come from The Good Shepherd Home. Here, there is no ignorance between the normal people and the crippled. Wheelchairs are taken for granted. They are forgotten. That is the way the general public should look upon them."

There is a tendency among people unassociated with cripples to look down upon them as children—all of them children.

But then again, there is a tendency for the crippled to wrap themselves in a false coat of pride and self-consciousness.

"I've got an answer to this—so simple you might think it foolish. The answer is to get to know each other.

"We can encourage you just as you have encouraged us. We can help to fight diseases, birth injuries and other forces that cripple the body just as you do. The experience we have is as valuable as the learned books of doctors.

"With God's help, we will conquer the meaning of the words *invalid*, *crippled* and *handicapped*. But we must do it together—you the strong in body and willing and we the weak in body but strong in experience and knowledge of crippled limbs."

Good heavens, who was filling the impressionable mind of twenty-one-year-old Carl with such radical ideas? Ramps? Federal laws? Elevators? Understanding? What next?

Carl is fifty-nine in this eightieth anniversary year. He has college degrees, a college-educated wife Rowena who is also in a wheelchair, normal children, a long pedigree of titles, honors and awards, a career in rehabilitation that has been served almost entirely at Good Shepherd.

He's the most delightfully irreverent writer ever to grace the pages of *Sweet Charity*. If someone does a book on "The Humor of Good Shepherd," half the material will be his old stuff. Who else still talks about the old trolley car days on St. John Street and how you could really zip down the street if you got a wheel of your wheelchair into a groove of the trolley track?

He was in graduate school when he married Rowena.

Connie noted to the Good Shepherd board in September 1961 that Carl, a Home boy and also a teacher at the Home, was on leave of absence, studying for a master's degree at the University of Southern Illinois.

"Last year, we gave him a grant of $100 a month to assist in his education. Fritz is married now. The girl he married is also on a wheelchair.

"In view of the fact that nobody really believes two can live as cheaply as one, I recommend we increase his grant to $150 a month for the duration of his school work, which will be until May 1962."

The board agreed.

Carl's still full of challenging ideas.

He says Good Shepherd was doing concepts of approach to the real needs of persons with disabilities long before the eggheads and other folks from the ivory towers discovered some of them.

"A great deal of emphasis in today's approach relates around normalization . . . that people should be treated not as exceptional, but just as people.

"We were practicing this long before others began to think of de-institutionalizing disabled people."

To Carl, Good Shepherd has been more of a community than anything else . . . with a larger number of people with a physical problem than you'd find on the streets.

One of the things he appreciated the most was the lack of structure. What has been done at Good Shepherd was done because it was natural . . . and because it was right.

Carl felt a responsibility to Good Shepherd and to himself. It was a privilege to be there. He didn't have the right to expect he'd be given anything.

"The Good Shepherd Home is dealing in the cutting edge of all the changes that are taking place . . . theories . . . approaches . . . debates about things that didn't exist when I was a kid.

"Yet, some of these things were here then, just because it made good sense."

Wasn't that something Papa said, that The Good Shepherd Home had to be run with a good measure of common sense?

Growing up was not all fun. And some of the frustrations Carl experienced meant that the world would have to change. He couldn't go to the public school. He had to go to the Good Shepherd School because there was no mandate that a wheelchair student had to be accepted.

"We had to take our anger and vent it in a constructive way," Carl says. "Sure, there was a gulf between the able-bodied and the handicapped. They were the normals and we were the cripples. That's the way we referred to each other, but we didn't group that way.

"When it came to chasing the gals—on a social level—the differences became apparent.

"Growing up here was a good experience. It taught me reality. It was a real world. It wasn't sheltered. There was never a fence around the place.

"By the grace of God, The Good Shepherd Home was ahead of the times it was in. We never saw the wisdom of what we were doing."

He finds in Connie Raker a special human being who has a sense of the life of the disabled.

"All the guys who made it from The Good Shepherd Home were the mean little types, not the lovable docile Tiny Tims. We usually caused Connie more trouble than we were worth. We stayed out late. We were striving to express ourselves.

"If I had lived at home with my family and had not had the chance to develop socially and intellectually, I would not have been able to develop. I needed that freedom."

He shakes his head and says, "The things kids do . . ." Then, he mentions how he'd try to zip around backwards in his wheelchair.

All the people employed at Good Shepherd were simply referred to as "workers." That, too, was a reflection of the freedom at Good Shepherd.

The place had huge festivals in the summer. The alumni would do a lot of the arranging, booking acts, doing public relations. It was an exciting time. The alums used a lot of the money raised to sponsor a basketball team in the city leagues. And the wheelchair residents would go to the games in an open truck in January.

The kids are gone. It's all adults.

Sometimes during Carl's years, Good Shepherd had whole families living here—the mother would work as a cook and the father as a fireman.

"There isn't a person in my memory who had potential who wasn't supported and helped. I can't think of one who gave a damn about himself that someone else didn't care about, too," he says.

Carl arrived after Papa Raker's death. But he knew Mama well. He says she was a great Democrat who was up on politics. They'd hold mock elections and have heated discussions in the dining room. Carl was always the radical. He and Mama thought alike.

Shortly after her death in August 1962, Carl wrote a beautiful eulogy of her.

While there were no fences around Good Shepherd, there was that eight-inch curb.

Carl took his high school training at the Good Shepherd School with teachers brought in by Allentown High principal Clifford "Chips" Bartholomew.

But in 1973, Carl founded Operation Overcome because the school district was going to put up a new high school science lab that would not be wheelchair accessible. And the Pennsylvania Department of Labor and Industry let it go by.

"We got ourselves a lawyer. The result was the school district put in an elevator. That was really the making of Operation Overcome. Good Shepherd was and is the meeting place for the organization.

"Allentown has responded well so far."

Recalling a battle that same year over the new Hamilton Mall in downtown Allentown seems to bring Carl a special joy.

The broad purpose was to make the public aware of the architectural barriers that needlessly restrict the handicapped. It was spearheaded by staff and guests at Good Shepherd.

As *Sweet Charity* quoted Carl at the time, many handicapped people live alone. They make modifications to their homes and cars so they can live independently. It's a matter of pride that they can manage without always having to call upon someone else to help them.

Once away from a familiar dwelling, they are confronted with a maze of architectural barriers often unnoticed by their unrestricted peers—curbs, steps, the narrow booths with telephones placed high out of reach, the impassable restroom enclosures and the awkward-to-pass-through doors and entrances.

"We don't feel architects and planners are our enemies," Carl said at the time. "Often, they are simply not aware of the barriers we are talking about. We want to make it evident that such barriers can be inexpensively avoided in construction and often easily eradicated where they now exist."

Carl was director of vocational rehabilitation at Good Shepherd in that era. Helping lead the campaign were Morris Blinderman, vice president of the Four Leaf Clover Club, an Allentown civic organization of handicapped persons, and Delores "Shookie" Shook, social program director at Good Shepherd. All three had been longtime residents at the Home.

There had been a state law on the books since 1967 requiring schools, hospitals and public buildings receiving state and federal support to be built with appropriate consideration for handicapped persons.

One of Carl's pet peeves concerned the new Hamilton Mall. During the planning stages, he urged the city's Redevelopment Authority to place ramps intermittently along curb lines or bevel the curbs so a motorized wheelchair could maneuver them.

The authority dropped the curbs from eight inches to four inches. It was like reducing the number of steps from eight to four. It did no good. Carl fumed.

William Scharf, director of Allentown's Department of Community Development, said access to the mall for the handicapped was considered in the planning.

Hadn't the authority lowered the curbs, installed laybys for passenger cars to discharge people and made islands on the north and south sides of the Center Square monument level with the street.

Scharf hid behind the architect in saying that the authority decided against having tailored ramps or indentations on his advice. The concern was safety of all the public, Scharf claimed.

"We feared that someone walking normally might not know about the ramps and might slip and fall on an icy, sloped surface. Ramps could also cause a snow-removal problem for plows. We wanted something that would work well for all the people.

"Besides, we had the impression that most handicapped people are accompanied by someone else anyway."

Ray Crissey, director of the Good Shepherd Rehabilitation Hospital, jumped all over that reasoning. Sure, most handicapped people are accompanied, but that is because of architectural barriers. Without them, they could often maneuver by themselves.

Curbs of reduced height, for example, make it easier for a wheelchair to be lifted over the obstacles. But if the curbs were eliminated, the person could go it alone; and if people got used to the existence of strategically placed ramps, they would not be a safety hazard.

To show public officials the problem, Odhner and his colleagues organized a "Roll on the Mall" that July 18. "We want them to sit in our wheelchairs and see for themselves what we are up against," he said.

And they did—including the mayor, the candidates for mayor, the mall architect and a county commissioner. It was an extraordinary photo opportunity. The old message of Papa and Verna Hoppes was obviously getting around town.

Shookie told the gathering that "we are not advocating expensive alterations to buildings and streets. An inexpensive ramp could be placed over part of the steps when a building is being used. Even one or two steps make a building inaccessible."

But Carl recalls now that nothing really was done about this for months. And then the next thing was that Governor Milton Shapp was coming in for the dedication.

"We threatened to picket. We wrote to the governor and told him why and, boy—zoom, zoom, zoom—those macadam ramps were put in."

Carl says the full measure of handicapped people having arrived will be "when you see a television commercial with a person in a wheelchair scrubbing his teeth."

Well, it has not quite come to that. But here in this spring of the eightieth anniversary year, a wheelchair athlete has made it on the cover of the Wheaties box. And *The Morning Call* carried three pictures of the winners of the Boston Marathon—the first male runner, the first female runner and the first wheelchair competitor.

Carl says, "The extent of disability is significantly increasing. Trauma units are scraping people off the highways. Young quadriplegics are coming into our rehabilitation hospital and they're gone in three or four weeks.

"What Good Shepherd does is enable people to continue their lives. Everybody is disabled sometime. That doesn't mean you give up living. What we sell is functional living. That's the message we are giving."

Good Shepherd serves hundreds of people a day.

Raker Center has 135 residents. About eighty percent of Raker Center residents will be here for life. They're all adults. Their families are growing old and aren't able to care for them.

"I don't see that The Good Shepherd Home residential program will change its purpose. But in the future, there will also be individual living support for those able to go on to their own homes, support services—transportation, housing, adaptive devices— even for the most severely handicapped, a kind of self-help so they can retain control over their lives.

"There is the matter of education. Many with multiple physical disabilities also have learning disabilities.

"Then, there's what we call psycho-social development. Often, they've been over-protected, raised as children. They don't see themselves as an adequate person.

"Independent living skills—learning how to live with disability so you can function. Vocational—learning how to work."

He says that for some people mainstreaming is not the answer. What he mentions is something that Dale Sandstrom has been touting in recent years—what might be called a Good Shepherd Academy. It would include some kind of cooperative program with the public schools. "You don't want to segregate disabled people from the able-bodied."

Carl concludes, "This is still a caring place, where the history of the place kind of roams the halls like a ghost." ❖

There is an opportunity here
to move heaven and earth, if
this work is done right.

Sweet Charity
September-October 1933

The Good Shepherd Home was the Protestant work
ethic in action before anybody ever used the term.

The youngsters—and the oldsters—at Good
Shepherd Home had to work to the fullest of their
abilities from the day they arrived.

Viola Hunt, the first child, was expected to help.
After all, when she arrived in early 1908, there were
the two small Raker girls to help care for—four-year-
old Roberta and seven-year-old Ruth.

The same for Aunt Mary Eisenhard, the first of the
elderly who became a part of the Good Shepherd
family in November 1908. She was eighty, but she was
nonetheless called an associate, a helper—and that
was a condition on which all future residents were to
enter.

Early on, Papa Raker was saying he wanted his
orphans to become self-supporting . . . while all the
same conceding to *Sweet Charity* readers that
"crippled orphans and infant orphans are not a
profitable investment from the worldly financial
standpoint."

With the construction of a new laundry building in
1912, *Sweet Charity* reported that the second floor
would be for manual training purposes.

A speaker at the 1912 Anniversary Day, J.S. Herberling, noted that Fairview Cemetery Association donated a beautiful burial plot for those Good Shepherd children who will not survive their physical infirmities.

But what of those who do, despite perhaps being blind or crippled?

"I plead for someone to supply the means of enabling this Home to train these children to be self-supporting.

"These children must live. How well and how happily they live will depend on the intelligent preparation that is given them here for the years to come."

And it was a bright new manual training room on the second floor of the laundry that *Sweet Charity* readers saw in their July-August 1915 issue, with Papa and the boys posed at the work benches.

During the school year, the youngsters receive a lesson a week in that work shop under a competent teacher, the text explained. "During vacations, they spend their time on the farms and in the manual training rooms.

"With the public schools, religious instruction, manual training, farm work, truck patch, chores around the Home and farms and plenty of time to play, we are attempting to give our children the best advantages we can."

Papa could rarely resist a chance to brag: "We have been told that Central High School of Philadelphia does not have the manual training outfit the Home has."

Charles Krick and Ulysses Grembach of the Muhlenberg College Class of 1918 were instructing the boys in manual training.

A 1920 *Sweet Charity* hailed Pearl Irene Sweitzer who had spent ten years at the Home. The Home saw her through the grades and also high school, the first Home child to attend what was then the new Allentown High, plus courses in dressmaking and stenography. "She is now self-supporting," the Home announced with obvious pride.

242

And *Sweet Charity* readers were repeatedly shown the scene of the blind Eva Pauley at the typewriter.

On the other end of the age scale, when Dr. George Trabert and his wife Elizabeth, both in their eighties, arrived from Minneapolis in the mid-1920s, Dr. Trabert was quickly put to work.

In a large measure, he became Dr. Wackernagel's successor in ministering to the other elderly, performing baptisms and weddings and writing regularly for *Sweet Charity.*

In 1929, Papa seemed to envision an idea that Connie would later develop, expand and make one of the foundation walls of the entire Good Shepherd enterprise—the sheltered workshop.

Papa said many people will contribute to help the Home support crippled youngsters, secure braces for them and provide them with an education. But these same people will not employ the cripples when they are prepared for life's work.

He said that almost every crippled child has some God-given gift by which to make an honest living and do some good in the world. And most cripples are able to fight their own battles for independence.

But if they fail in their first attempt, Good Shepherd takes them back and prepares them anew for something they're better adapted for. Some are already making their third attempt.

"We see the need of a building for just such special cases and a workshop where proper employment can be given them."

A decade later, in the aftermath of a 1938 conference at Cleveland of the International Society for the Aid of the Crippled, Connie Raker was preaching the message of the sheltered workshop—first to the board and then to the public through the pages of *Sweet Charity.*

He had visited what was called the Sunbeam Shop in Cleveland—a large, well-lit building where disabled men and women worked.

"The men work in a well-equipped carpentry shop and make many useful and salable articles. The women work on sewing machines and do all phases of work with cloth," he reported.

The Sunbeam Shop got orders from hospitals from Cleveland to Chicago. The workers made gowns and masks worn by surgeons and nurses in operating rooms and the napkins surgical instruments were wrapped in.

"The Sunbeam Shop does a grand work which few other institutions in the country do. They give organized work to the handicapped," he exulted.

And then this twenty-six-year-old voiced some dreams for Good Shepherd:

"It is our earnest hope at The Good Shepherd Home that we will be able to have such a sheltered workshop. Then crippled men and women who now have no hope of employment in industry will be able to work and support themselves. They will then be able to rent small apartments near the Home and earn a living in the workshop.

"At present we have an occupational therapy shop where the boys and girls work two hours a day. Here on several looms, they are able to weave rugs, tapestry and handbags. Under the guidance of a trained worker, they make many useful articles.

"We hope that this occupational therapy shop may just be the beginning and that later we may have a well-regulated shop in which handicapped men and women can earn a living."

Connie got his dream and then some—but not right away.

He would renew his hopes to the board in early 1953—in the immediate aftermath of a nearly $400,000 addition to the main building for the disabled. That alone would mean a potential of forty more who might be trained for jobs, many definitely able to do something with their hands.

As he saw it, it was to be a workshop "for the handicapped within our gates." But it would also serve the handicapped out across the Lehigh Valley as well.

There were other sheltered workshops for the handicapped, like the one on Fourteenth Street in Manhattan run by the Federation for the Handicapped and the Binghamton, New York, Sheltered Workshop.

But this one at Good Shepherd would be the first anywhere tied to an existing institution. There would be no need, for instance, for a cafeteria, because the Home was right there with its own kitchen. In fact, the kitchen in the new wing of the main building had deliberately been built to accommodate more than the resident population.

The existing small shop was already too small, Connie said. He recommended a simple factory loft-type construction—an office for the director and lavatories, the rest one large open room. Nothing fancy on the outside either.

"I am convinced there are concerns in the Lehigh Valley that would give us piecework, which would keep many handicapped people employed," Connie said in his report to the board.

"For instance, Rodale Electric Co. in Emmaus makes many electrical appliances which some of our handicapped men and women could assemble quite easily. As a matter of fact, our boys and girls did this type of work during the war."

Connie contended that many handicapped people then living home-bound lives could have a real sense of usefulness. They could pay their own way. With transportation to the workshop, some could live with their families.

Also, it would not be impossible in the future for some of these handicapped families to rent houses in the neighborhood. The houses directly across Fifth Street would lend themselves to this kind of living because of the absence of steps.

They would not be admitted to The Good Shepherd Home, but they would still become part of the Good Shepherd community. "They could go to our chapel, attend our movies and all our functions, yet be independent, self-supporting individuals," he said.

He put a cost figure of $20,000 on the building.

And what he had suggested anew came amid a major change in direction for Good Shepherd. The care of physically normal children was being phased out. It was something that had been mulled over for a long time. It was part of what was happening in the nation—the disappearance of the orphanage, in part because of tougher (and expensive) government requirements on living quarters, in part because such children were being placed more and more in foster homes.

Connie got in touch with a parent or other responsible relative of the normal children in the cottages. Some were making arrangements. Others simply didn't reply.

By early 1954, that operation had been completed. The few who remained were transferred to the main building, and the room in the cottages meant space for fifteen more elderly.

But that was limited, too, by regulations. The cottages had no elevators. Thus, only the ambulatory aged could be housed there.

Sweet Charity readers were greeted with a sketch of the workshop on the cover of the July-August 1955 issue. Appropriately, the drawing included a man with crutches.

And on the first page inside the magazine was a blaring headline **JOBS WANTED!** and an article by Connie on his hopes for the sheltered workshop.

He cited Harold, a polio victim living with his brother twenty miles north of Allentown. With his wheelchair, he got around well enough on the first floor at home. But other than occasional rides with his brother, he seldom got out of the house.

Though Harold was paralyzed from the waist down, his one hand was all right, the other only slightly touched with paralysis.

Harold's brother worked at Bethlehem Steel Co. and drove right by Good Shepherd on his way to work. So there would be little trouble to transport Harold to and from work. Good Shepherd attendants would teach the brother ways to make it easier to get Harold in and out of the car.

Here, for the first time, Harold will have the glorious satisfaction of knowing he is carrying his own weight, paying his own way.

Connie asked: "If the average physically sound individual needs the feeling of accomplishment his job gives him for a sense of well-being, how much more does the handicapped?

"This is the way The Good Shepherd Home is trying to solve the unemployment problem for a group of very willing and able but until now overlooked workers—the physically handicapped."

And if the ones Good Shepherd trains and employs do so well that they can go out into industry, the Home will gladly shove them out the door as quickly as possible to positions in offices and plants.

The issue of *Sweet Charity* was filled with page after page of pictures of handicapped people at work at machines at that Binghamton Sheltered Workshop.

Connie probably didn't look upon himself as a civil rights champion for the physically handicapped. But that's what he was —and is.

He appealed to *Sweet Charity* readers for help in this as in anything else at Good Shepherd.

It was the loving thing to do. While the workshop would be operated on a nonprofit basis, providing for the plant and equipment would take money from unselfish people. It was also the wise thing to do economically.

Sweet Charity proclaimed: "No degree of economic gain can measure the social and moral satisfaction obtained by the successfully employed handicapped worker and his family. Nor is it possible to measure the value to society of the transformation of these individuals from dependents to productive self-reliant persons."

As the workshop neared, the board organized a workshop committee involving several board members and people from industry in the community.

At both workshops Connie visited, the greatest amount of work was done in electronics. So Good Shepherd called upon Fred Hanson, then head of the Allentown works of Western Electric, to assist in the project.

The opening of the workshop was set for February 21, 1958, to the day the fiftieth anniversary of the arrival of Viola Hunt as the first child to come under the care of The Good Shepherd Home. There was to be a banquet with Henry Viscardi as the guest speaker. Viscardi was founder and president of Abilities Inc., which employed only the handicapped at its plant on Long Island.

But the biggest snowstorm of the year hit on dedication day, and the program had to be canceled. The dedication would have to await the Fiftieth Anniversary Pilgrimage that June.

Meanwhile, life at the workshop was getting underway with the immediate goal the employment of twenty-five people under workshop manager Bernard L. Gilbert. Connie reported at the outset that contracts had already been arranged with several industrial firms in the Allentown area for the workshop to produce component parts for electronic equipment and for other purposes.

Late in the year, Connie lamented to the board that the workshop was progressing slowly. "We probably began the work at the worst possible time. The recession has prevented him from getting orders for work," Connie wrote.

People in industry who promised the workshop subcontracts unfortunately, when contacted, said they had just laid off some of their regular workers.

The workshop also had to deal with an unfounded rumor that it was hiring people off the street, handicapped or not. That was squelched when Good Shepherd had both labor and management representatives from Allentown's General Electric plant come and see for themselves. They went away impressed.

This slow start, though, would explain the prolonged silence in *Sweet Charity* about how the project was doing.

But by May 1959, Connie was pleased to report that the workshop was showing very substantial progress. He said the day was soon coming when fifty people would be employed there. Its workforce was ten.

Things really started moving in the spring of 1960 when 150 business leaders from the Allentown area were invited to a dinner, a talk by Fred Hanson of Western Electric on the workshop and then a tour of the facility.

And it was quite a pitch they got from Hanson. "When we employ the services of The Good Shepherd Workshop, we do more than just help give jobs to the handicapped," he said to the assemblage. "We give the handicapped an opportunity to use their available talents and become self-sufficient.

"They are ready to work—if we will just put the tools into their hands."

Newspaper Editor William D. Reimert was master of ceremonies. Catholic Priest Theodore Heineman gave the invocation and Rabbi William Greenburg pronounced the benediction.

The occasion was a tremendous success. One result was that the manufacturers' division of the Chamber of Commerce wanted to take the workshop under its wing.

The added attention even attracted some patient at the Allentown State Hospital who wrote to Connie:

"I read in the paper a few days ago that you are planning to enlarge the workshop. I would like to have a little corner, a few square feet, to continue my experiments on citrus fruit pills which I have been doing the past ten years here in the state hospital in secret. I would like to come out in the open market to commercialize it."

In the most diplomatic terms, Connie wrote back that there were no openings at the workshop, that it was filled to capacity. He closed, "Trusting that everything will work out well for you, we pray that God will bless you richly in all your endeavors."

The workshop would soon be rechristened Unlimited Skills. And the word was getting around that it was quite a going operation. Pennsylvania Governor David Lawrence and author Pearl Buck of Bucks County—in Allentown for some other celebrated events—both showed up at the same time October 6, 1961, to view the workshop with Hanson, its advisory committee chairman. That visit put them on the cover of the next *Sweet Charity*. Hanson was one to enlist some formidable industrial and civic leaders to work with him. He gained new customers to ensure the continuity of the operation.

He added some general use machine tools, benches and facilities to broaden the range of production. He recruited volunteers from among area engineers to act as manufacturing consultants and established a policy that the shop would not become a prime manufacturing unit but would remain a subcontractor to others.

Connie had some haunting words about the workshop and a new project, a rehabilitation center, for *Sweet Charity* readers in the summer of 1963. They came amid the first year the workshop was to finish in the black:

"If you could look into the future and see The Good Shepherd Home fifty years from now, we are convinced that two things for which it will be best known are the workshop for the handicapped, which currently is giving employment to thirty-five crippled men and women from the Lehigh Valley, and the rehabilitation center which now is only on paper."

Well, we're only half way from 1963 to 2013. But those words look pretty good, if an evaluation at the halfway point is permitted.

With the growth of the workshop came the need for more space. By 1969, the number of employees had grown as Connie envisioned. And total business was the best in its eleven-year history—despite the fact that its biggest supplier, General Electric, had been on strike most of the last quarter.

Connie recalls that every time he passed a one-story building at Lehigh and Vultee Streets he'd tell himself that building was built for Good Shepherd. "It was wheelchair accessible from day one. There wasn't a step in the place. I said: We must buy this." And when the building became available—around 1970—Good Shepherd did buy it.

Here in this eightieth anniversary year, that location thrives with work. It is now known as Good Shepherd Industrial Services.

Yet, it was not the listing of the products assembled or the pedigree of workshop advisory board members that told the story so well as it was yarns about the people involved. Tom McNabb of Allentown was a case in point.

With his white hair and his gentle face, he looked like everybody's kindly grandfather. He had had a lengthy and successful career running a machine business in Allentown that made machines for other companies.

And, like a lot of people, somehow he got involved with Good Shepherd. Often he found himself redesigning or rebuilding a wheelchair or some other special device for someone at the Home. Tools and machinery were frequently lent to the Home.

And when the Good Shepherd workshop came along in 1958, Tom was one of the first to join its advisory committee. With the passing of his wife in 1964, he sold his business and soon transferred his skills and energies to the workshop as a volunteer.

He was a regular at 8 a.m. for years at the workshop, staying until at least early afternoon. He did most of the repairs on the shop's machinery and tools. He determined the cost for new tooling and often designed and built the fixtures and tools needed for new jobs.

From the time he was a youngster he read biographies. "But few biographies have taught or inspired me like the people I daily encounter at The Good Shepherd Workshop," he once told *Sweet Charity*.

"Far from being depressing, the exact opposite is true when working with these people. Their determination, will power, enthusiasm and sincere appreciation for whatever you do for them has a unique way of rubbing off on you. You think you are helping them, but, actually, they are helping you far more."

One of the success stories of the workshop was that it shoved its top workers out the door. It mainstreamed them into jobs in business and industry.

The old workshop at South Fifth Street has undergone a substantial transformation and expansion just in this eightieth anniversary year. It is now the Robert and Marian Edwards Center, named in behalf of

251

a board member and his wife from Slatington whose $750,000 gift to the endowment fund made the expansion possible. It was the largest lifetime gift Good Shepherd ever received.

One entranceway has the words "Industrial Medicine" over the door. The other says "Vocational Services."

Here, in the industrial medicine program, workers injured in job-related accidents are tested, retrained and toughened with the goal of being sent back to work. As of early 1988, some twenty-eight companies had contracted with Good Shepherd for this service.

It saves the insurance companies money by getting the employees back to work quicker. It's a project that has really taken off.

There is a cab of a Mack truck among the equipment where a client can simulate various moves in a vehicle.

And there is what's called a BTE, standing for Baltimore Therapeutic Equipment. It's a standup contraption with a lot of possible attachments. One attachment may require the individual to practice the motions necessary for operating a screwdriver, another to simulate sawing, yet another to push or pull.

The other section of the Edwards Building, Good Shepherd Vocational Services, is to test new handicapped people to see what abilities they have for possible job placement. This includes determining skills in working computers.

Meanwhile, at the sheltered workshop on Lehigh Street, Thomas Stenhouse, vice president for Good Shepherd Industrial Services, says the mission now is much more challenging than when the workshop started. The shop has to try to deal with the acutely disabled.

Many of the so-called handicapped of twenty years ago, who would have worked in the shop, are today finding places for themselves in society and in the regular business world. These would be people like paraplegics in wheelchairs whose bodies from the waist up are normal.

Tom says that even with the severely disabled, they

have to be able to do the work or out they go. "They're trained to understand the business world." He says there's no toleration for the idea that the world owes you a living.

Besides the severely handicapped, deaf and blind people, the workshop also deals closely with organizations serving those with language disabilities, people with drug and alcohol problems, prison release, probation board and a farm workers association.

Tom says the workshop needs the support of those agency people to offset the lack of productivity by the severely handicapped.

In the earlier years, many handicapped people were productive and were not low-functioning. Fortunately, a lot of those people were placed in employment in the community.

But as Tom points out, "The low functioning are still to be cared for. That's our mission, and we'll always be in that position. We depend on those few productive people to make up the difference between what would normally be produced and what is actually produced."

The Lehigh Street facility puts labels and addresses on mass mailings and also handles mail distribution. It vacuum packs products in plastic, then shrinks and blister packs them. It performs microfilming services. It has a quick copy division, capable of turning out 14,000 items an hour printed on both sides. It has a print shop, a machine shop and an electromechanical assembly section.

The plant also has the largest paper recycling station in the Lehigh Valley—handling a million pounds of paper a month as of 1988.

Tom has been with the workshop since 1970. He had never worked with people with handicaps before, but had been giving them work as a subcontractor for a number of years before that through his own company in Easton.

"I really didn't know why Tom Stenhouse was saying yes to the position," he says. "But I really feel God had a plan for me, and He did. When I see these people with their disabilities, I still think I'm a very fortunate man."

It was a social atmosphere when he first arrived, with twenty workers sitting around in squares talking about what they did the night before.

What really made the workshop take off was that Tom gave them more difficult tasks and they responded. Papa Raker had an old line: "The more you expect the more you are likely to get." And Tom was proving that with the people in the workshop.

"They were capable of much, much more, and they were earning more. They loved that. We hired more staff. We soon ran out of room."

The workshop leased more space. Then, it bought the building on Lehigh Street. Today, counting several satellite locations, it occupies 95,000 square feet of floor space.

In Tom's first year, with twenty people, the workshop gross was around $180,000. This latest year, with 250 workers, the gross is around $4 million.

Tom says there are many frustrations in this endeavor.

Probably the one that hit him the most when he first arrived was in going from the regular run of the mill industry where everybody worked at 90-110 percent of capacity to entering a field where people were working at 20, 60, 100 percent with all kinds of disabilities. "It was quite a change, at least to me," he says.

The joy of heading the workshop "is just being here to serve the Lord in this capacity," Tom says. "It's a God-given gift to work with these people and see them progressing, enjoying their work."

Now, to find some Good Shepherd workers supervised out in the community, you have to turn to a separate vocational services program. In 1987, Good Shepherd Vocational Services placed 102 physically, mentally and emotionally challenged people in jobs.

Louise Wagner, who teaches sign language to a lot of people, runs a Good Shepherd crew at Pennsylvania Power & Light Co. in downtown Allentown that opens and sorts 100,000 to 150,000 payments a week. Good Shepherd has had the contract for this for nine years.

This "Projects With Industry" program has attracted the attention of the Harvard Business Review.

There is a crew of thirteen, each with a disability of some kind. "You have to have a lot of dexterity to do the job," Louise says. This is part-time work, eighteen to twenty hours a week.

Each worker is handling a check and receipt stub every four seconds on assembly-line machines. Those receipts can go in any one of eight categories.

"Not every disabled person could do it. Not every disabled person who comes on will make it. It's tedious, the same thing every day. Your eyes get tired. Your back gets tired. It involves getting up early in the morning."

Two of the crew start at 6 a.m., the rest at 6:30. They're all responsible for their own transportation.

Louise says when PP&L raises rates or has some problem with nuclear power, then there are notes with the bills—some of them X-rated.

Across these nine years, Louise has supervised about 150 employees. Some have moved on to full-time PP&L jobs. Others have gone to full-time jobs elsewhere.

Just west of Allentown, another Good Shepherd crew is at work for Aetna Insurance Co., here dealing with the opening of mail regarding claims.

At PP&L, the Good Shepherd people operate in a room of their own. With Aetna, they are ten people in one segment of a massive room that has dozens of other Aetna employees. And the regular Aetna workers have included the Good Shepherd crew in such things as office Christmas festivities.

Good Shepherd staff member Kathy Wolf says this started in early 1987 with two people helping out in the mailroom. It just blossomed out.

This program involves working primarily with people with chronic mental illness. "You're helping people realize their potential—to push them a little bit in something they may have been frightened of," she says.

When an individual works at one job and gains some confidence, that person can move up to the next level. Three in the project have already moved on to regular jobs with Aetna within the first year.

And beyond these supervised jobs are the Good Shepherd alumni who are out of there on their own—like Kenneth "Wheels" McHenry of Cherryville, who at fifty has been out in the world with his wheelchair for a generation . . . with a job at AT&T, a marriage, an attractive one-story home in a quiet community and a zany modified motorcycle that he can drive while seated in his wheelchair. He even has a neighbor down the street in a wheelchair. ❖

It is only a question of time
when The Good Shepherd
Home must have its own
hospital.

Sweet Charity
March-April 1912

A rehabilitation hospital on the Good Shepherd
grounds was long a dream, an obsession, with Connie
Raker. And it has become a reality to such an extent
that the name Good Shepherd is known far and wide
for what it does to take battered bits of humanity,
shape them back into functioning and often productive
individuals and then send them back into the real
world again.

There are items here and there in some of the early
issues of *Sweet Charity* that indicate that perhaps
Papa had given Connie some gentle nudges in the
direction of a rehabilitation hospital.

Besides the quote at the head of this chapter, there
were:

Dr. H.H. Hart, director of the Child Helping
Department of the Russell Sage Foundation of New
York, said at the seventh anniversary in 1915 that
Good Shepherd would soon need an orthopedic
hospital to properly care for its crippled children.

Dr. George Gebert of Tamaqua, before his tenure as
board president, addressed the 1919 Anniversary Day
gathering about a hospital:

"One great drawback is keenly felt by the board—the lack of hospital facilities. Superintendent Raker took a number of the boys to Philadelphia for examination. Some were operated on and helped to the extent of being able to walk with braces.

"But a hospital should be right on the grounds."

Dr. Gebert, soon after he became board president, renewed that message in *Sweet Charity* in 1925. The topic of his article was the board's plans for the aged. And while he admitted he was to confine his writing to that topic, he just couldn't resist throwing in a brief pitch for an orthopedic hospital. The hospital was a large factor waiting and wanting, he said.

"The board is conscious of the truth that God knows the need and will put it into the heart of some of His beneficiaries to respond to the call."

Sweet Charity in the summer of 1934 reported that the general health of the guests had been good during the previous winter.

"Of course, this spring some of our children had to join in the general epidemic of measles which spread over Allentown. Whenever we have any serious cases of illness, the Allentown and Sacred Heart hospitals offer their services free to our guests."

In September 1937, Dr. Morgan Person of Allentown was winding up his first year as a doctor and just about his first full year of volunteer service to The Good Shepherd Home.

His work for Good Shepherd included eighty-two visits to the Home, eight patients sent to the hospital for various ailments, twenty-two injections and one circumcision performed.

The total cost was $48. His services were entirely given in the name of charity.

He offered a few suggestions to the board in a single-spaced four-page letter that was treasured enough to be preserved in the Good Shepherd files for fifty years.

His first proposal was an annual physical examination of each guest.

Next, this young doctor recommended that Good Shepherd establish a dispensary and furnish it with the essential instruments and equipment needed to meet the fundamental requirements of good medical care.

"This will eliminate the possibility of equipment and medicines not being on the premises when so needed. In addition, a dispensary will give a definite sense of security to all in official position against possible future criticism from lay persons and the Department of Welfare," Dr. Person wrote.

He also suggested budgeting $500 a year for medical care—beyond the nurse-matrons already on duty. He suggested $260 of that as an annual retainer for the doctor and the rest for medicines and supplies for the dispensary. That retainer was only about a third of usual charges, he said. It was far less than the cost at homes that sheltered children in full possession of all faculties.

He had it broken down to cost per patient: "Don't you gentleman think it is a small price to pay at only $6.60 per guest for insurance against any medical or surgical condition that might arise in the future?"

A retainer for the physician would make that individual a definite part of the official Good Shepherd family, he said. It would recognize that the health and physical care of the children is on an equal plane with their spiritual, moral and mental care. And it would enable the Home to report to the Department of Public Welfare that it had a part-time physician on a salary basis.

"Lastly, it would make the physician, in return, more responsible, give him a sense of security, not to mention the fact that he would no longer be led to think he was given less consideration and payment than the plumber, carpenter or even the janitor."

The board bought it.

Secretary Wahrmann replied that it was his privilege as well as duty to read Person's letter at the September board meeting.

First, Wahrmann said, the board extended its thanks for all Dr. Person had done in the past year. Next, it approved an honorarium of $22.50 a month ($270 a year) for him for the coming year. And, finally, it authorized the establishment of a dispensary and would seek donations for it.

—In September 1938, the Home dedicated a renovated workers building on South Sixth Street that included a dispensary. The room was furnished with supplies and equipment by a $500 donation from the Allentown District Luther League. Atty. Henry V. Scheirer, a past president of the State Luther League, gave the dedicatory address.

There was also a place for dental quarters figured in.

—Like his father a decade earlier, Connie Raker in the first 1943 *Sweet Charity* devoted his entire message to praise of Allentown Hospital, chief surgeon Robert Schaeffer, superintendent George Sherer and the entire staff for the way they had cared for patients from Good Shepherd.

"Our children and aged people received the best possible care. They could not have been cared for better if they had been paying guests in private rooms," Connie said.

"The Allentown Hospital is doing a Christian service, not only in caring for the medical and surgical needs of the crippled and aged of The Good Shepherd Home, but in the greater work it does for the entire community.

"To Allentown Hospital, we say: May the Lord continue to bless you in His work."

* * *

Longtime Home resident Morris Blinderman had an exciting new watchword—physio-therapy—to expound upon in 1949 for those like himself who were physically handicapped.

"The word spells new hope and possible realization of dreams of rehabilitation, dreams that may have been given up for lost by the easily discouraged," Blinderman told the *Sweet Charity* audience.

It was now the name of a new department, headed by registered nurse Eva Deibert, who was also instructor of student nurses in massage and exercise at Allentown Hospital. And in this Good Shepherd work, she quickly found herself engulfed in the lives of those she served. It was a blessed affliction that beset many normals who came for a job and wound up immersed in a loving career instead.

Blinderman wrote, "She has inspired in her patients a great determination to face the pain and discomfort of necessary operations, patience and courage in taking the first steps and to continue the hardships of learning to walk after a lifetime of sitting in a wheelchair and a deep willingness by her charges to face anything and do almost anything to gain physical progress and freedom."

Blinderman saw good reasons for this new department, reasons perhaps as deeply emblazoned upon his heart and mind as upon other physically handicapped people being helped . . . the driving will to walk, to overcome physical difficulties . . . the burning dreams of a more complete life and career . . . the will to explore the outside life and experiences of ordinary people and to become a part of all of it.

Physical therapy was not something new at Good Shepherd. It had been practiced in a less formal way for forty years there. Papa Raker possessed a keen determination to rehabilitate every crippled child or adult if possible and to spare no means in doing it, Blinderman said.

For specialized care, some had been taken to a famed orthopedic surgeon in Philadelphia, to the orthopedic clinic at Allentown Hospital or the State Crippled Children Hospital at Elizabethtown in Lancaster County.

Just look at the alumni who are well-stationed despite their handicaps—teachers, office workers, store clerks, governmental workers, craftsmen, factory help to mention just a few. Quite a number of crippled former guests married and raised families.

Blinderman said it was the Rev. Conrad W. Raker who was carrying on the cause of physical reconstruction, who inspired the establishment of the new quarters for this work. And it was his fond dream someday to have a warm exercising pool to bring out the best in weakened muscles of all victims of paralysis.

Three prominent orthopedic surgeons were working

with the young crippled guests—Drs. Richard White and Kenneth Weston of Allentown and Hahnemann hospitals and Dr. Joseph Reno, a surgeon for several hospitals and the Lehigh Valley Crippled Children's Society.

"Their tribute is renewed bodies and lives," Blinderman said.

Time was much a factor. The eagerness to overcome handicaps makes the patient impatient for results.

Nurse Deibert cautioned, "It must not be expected that after a few months of treatments these boys and girls can spring up and walk—as most of them have been disabled for several years, if not for life. In several months time, a number of them have been relieved of cumbersome braces and are beginning to use their limbs again."

Dr. White recalls, "Kenny Weston led me to Good Shepherd with all those kids with their cockeyed feet and cockeyed legs. He asked me to come in and straighten a few legs, that I could do it. Nobody knew how to brace them.

"It was a great place to work, a goldmine for experience, being able to help somebody if you knew what to do."

The covers of *Sweet Charity* were undergoing a bit of change in line with the physical therapy. There were pictures of young people learning to walk with the aid of parallel bars or a walker.

*   *   *

The September-October 1951 cover brought the first of a new generation of handicapped youngsters who would be outfitted in rather marvelous ways with legs and arms for ones they didn't have.

Her name was Marlene Cook. She was born without legs.

She came to the attention of the Home in 1942 through Rev. John Alberti of Philadelphia. Marlene was born to a member of his congregation, St. Paul's German Lutheran in Olney.

Connie visited her and was struck by her beauty.

262

"The child's face is perfect and shows a great deal of intelligence," he reported to the board. Her left hand was abnormal. But the main thing was her two feet seemed to come right out of the buttocks. Connie could see what problems a child of this kind could be for a one-parent family.

Marlene was nine months old when she arrived at Good Shepherd. She stayed until she was nineteen.

"My mother often told me that I would have sat in a chair if I hadn't gone to The Good Shepherd Home," says Marlene (Cook) Dundore in this eightieth anniversary year.

Marlene says she grew up without the love of her parents. Unlike many others, she saw the workers at Good Shepherd as people who didn't show love. Connie's reports on her to the board conveyed Marlene's feelings of rejection in such a way that the heartache seemed as much his as Marlene's.

Then, too, Marlene admits, "I was a brat. I talked back a lot. Often, I said I had a chip on my shoulder."

For all her inner turmoil, Marlene represented a heart-tugging story to *Sweet Charity* readers. Connie Raker sent her to the Kessler Institute at West Orange, New Jersey, where it was determined she could be fitted for legs, then to a hospital in Newark for an operation and then back to Kessler.

At age thirteen, when she was measured for her legs, she was asked: "How tall do you want to be?"

Marlene answered, "Five feet four."

And there was Marlene in the mid-1950s, twice the centerspread of *Sweet Charity* with before and after pictures of her and the legs, representing some of the new directions in which Good Shepherd was heading.

And Marlene would be one of the first to train at the state's new vocational rehabilitation center in Johnstown in 1960. Her course was in office procedures. She returned to Good Shepherd to become full-time switchboard operator in the Administration Building.

Those legs, unfortunately, didn't work out. Marlene says she got started with them too late, that she had abandoned them even before she left Good Shepherd for marriage and a family. "I felt trapped in them," she says.

Marlene, divorced, lives with a grown daughter now. She gets around in a car and a wheelchair. She says she's very happy. Much of her daily life is spent proselytizing for Jehovah's Witnesses, and her friends almost totally come from that group.

"I was glad I was raised at The Good Shepherd Home," Marlene says. And she recalls Mama Raker as a loving person—"though I probably didn't think so at the time."

* * *

Marlene used to pal around with Billy Anderson at Good Shepherd. "Bill and I were like brother and sister," she says.

Billy arrived at age twelve from Morgantown, West Virginia, in late 1954, a boy born without arms and with practically no legs. He had a sense of humor and a quick smile. He was bright. He was even rather mobile in a low four-wheel walker.

"His parents are obviously quite poor, but they have done very well in raising him to be a self-reliant young fellow," Connie said to the board.

Surgical and post-operative work on Billy would be staggering. And in the case of most artificial legs, good arms are needed for the use of crutches and for balance. Billy was without that necessary support.

Connie concluded, "It is impossible to say with any assurance that he will ever be made completely self-sufficient, but we can try."

Within five years of his arrival, Billy Anderson was being hailed as the outstanding achievement orthopedically in the life of The Good Shepherd Home. By then, he had been to both the Kessler Institute and the Institute for the Crippled and Disabled in New York City.

He had been equipped with legs of conventional design. But his arms operated on a totally new principle. They were powered by carbon-dioxide gas. Billy was wearing and demonstrating a pilot model.

He could pick up and eat a hamburger with the new arm, something impossible with the claw hand he had before.

Because he was such a pleasant, intelligent and friendly lad, he became a favorite of the people at the various institutes and agencies that had contact with him. Billy was sent to demonstrate the new arm at a meeting of physicians in Atlantic City and also before the Vocational Rehabilitation Council in Washington, D.C.

Connie at one point quipped that Billy has a career just in going around demonstrating the arm.

*   *   *

And it was shortly in the aftermath of these dramatic efforts with Marlene and Billy that Connie revealed his dreams for a rehabilitation center. He was as transparent as Papa when it came to really wanting something for Good Shepherd.

Connie's message in the September-October 1961 *Sweet Charity* was filled with exultation:

"Now a vacant lot . . . soon a modern rehabilitation center. The joy of creating something from nothing is a godlike pleasure the entire Good Shepherd Home staff is enjoying.

"We look forward to next spring when ground will be broken, but now we are reveling in the thrill of planning a building after our heart's desire."

That vacant lot at the southeast corner of Sixth and St. John has only been elevated to the status of paved parking lot for many of the staff at Good Shepherd. It was scrapped as the site for the rehab center, in part because it would have put a part of the Good Shepherd complex on the other side of wide and busy St. John Street from the rest of the buildings.

But the idea of a rehabilitation center did become a reality—in the center of the complex.

It is the building with the Twenty-third Psalm printed around the top. A visitor in this eightieth Anniversary year can't see all of the psalm by walking around the outside anymore. The psalmist's words on

the eastern end have been covered over by the new
fourth floor of the rehabilitation hospital, the latest
expansion of Good Shepherd's massive rehabilitation
program. But the missing words of the psalm have
been written again on a facing wall on the fourth floor
inside the hospital.

It took a couple years more than Connie originally
envisioned to build the rehab center. But that was
because he was telling everyone involved to take their
time, to do it carefully. His approach to the staff
members was: If you were building the ideal
rehabilitation center, what would you put in it? "And
that's what we built," he says.

This was also a project that involved Hill-Burton
funds, a program of matched money between the state
and federal government for hospitals. It meant
government supplying a third of the estimated
$707,000 cost of the building.

Dr. Samuel E. Kidd, president of the Eastern
Pennsylvania Synod, the successor to the old
Ministerium, saw Good Shepherd on a Hill-Burton list
for nearly $236,000. Pointing to the fact that synod's
parent denomination hadn't taken a position on Hill-
Burton funds, Kidd asked Connie to explain why the
Good Shepherd board applied.

In reply, Connie cited Lutheran institutions around
the country that had received Hill-Burton funds,
including $500,000 for Muhlenberg Medical Center
just a few miles away in Bethlehem.

One motivation, other than the actual financial help,
was that it would tie Good Shepherd closely in a
working relationship with many state and federal
agencies. "Many of these contacts are highly
beneficial," Connie said.

"For the first time, people in the Department of
Health, Education and Welfare in Washington and also
in Harrisburg know intimately the work the church is
doing for the physically handicapped at The Good
Shepherd Home."

He said the center wouldn't be the biggest in the
country, but one of the best.

Connie concluded, "We are really having a lot of fun

planning this venture. I am confident it will be the kind of thing Lutherans all over the world will point to with pride."

But even before ground was broken, Good Shepherd had assembled a rehabilitation team that already had accomplishments: Dr. Alfons J. Muller as medical director; Carl F. Odhner, rehabilitation counselor; Robert C. Zehner, chief physical therapist; Sara C. Steinberg, occupational therapist, and Dr. Albert L. Billig, psychologist.

Connie pointed to four particular patients:

The Rev. Gerald J. Jacoby of St. John's Lutheran, St. Johns, Luzerne County, a classmate of Connie's, who suffered a stroke December 15, 1963, that slightly involved his speech and paralyzed one side. The stroke had left him depressed.

At Connie's behest, he came for a month in the spring of 1964 to be worked on by the rehabilitation team. His progress was outstanding, particularly the lifting of his spirits.

Connie got in a bit of his own therapy for his old classmate. He had Pastor Jacoby read part of the Palm Sunday and Good Friday services, read the full service on Easter and then preach the following Sunday.

It was his first time in the pulpit since his stroke. "This was a real victory for him," Connie said.

Within a month, he returned to his parish.

Samuel Kospiah of Bethlehem, who lost his left leg from complications of diabetes, became the first amputee outpatient in February 1964. He came daily for gait training with his artificial leg, and that led to his return to work at a family market.

His presence marked the start of Good Shepherd as an amputee training center, able to accept patients from the State Bureau of Vocational Training.

There were also a spastic individual from a Presbyterian Church on Long Island, where Connie had preached, who spent two months at Good Shepherd for work evaluation and a gunshot victim who received daily treatments until he was able to return to work at Bethlehem Steel.

Even before the groundbreaking, Good Shepherd

already was serving eighteen outpatients.

Groundbreaking was set for June 28, 1964. The construction contract had been awarded to H.A. Williams Inc. at $683,000.

Four days before the ceremony, Phillipsburg attorney Henry Harms walked into the office and handed Connie $109,964 in securities from the Mabel K. Karchner estate.

After the necessary releases were signed, Harms said to Connie, "Do you know how Miss Karchner got to know about The Good Shepherd Home?"

Connie replied, "I have no idea."

Harms answered, "Through your speaking at St. John's in Easton."

The groundbreaking ceremony went perfectly. Pennsylvania's Public Welfare Secretary Arlin Adams told the 2,000 participants, "We maintain that the physical, mental, emotional and social needs of man are interdependent . . . the 'whole man' approach.

"The purpose of this center at The Good Shepherd Home will be to provide integrated rehabilitation services from the medical, vocational, psychological and social fields."

Connie's message was that "no event in our history—save the founding itself—is of such magnitude and importance." The center will provide the means to work with disabled persons on a better and larger scale.

At ninety-four, Rev. Wahrmann turned the first spade of earth.

The names of the initial medical staff were to appear in a glass case: Medical Director Alfons J. Muller, Dentist George E Jenkins and Doctors Clarence Holland, Robert H. Dilcher, Morton I. Silverman, Forrest G. Moyer, Richard K. White, Herman Meckstroth and Dominic Salines.

Afterward Connie noted, "The people of the community who actually make the wheels go were in attendance. Their presence was deeply appreciated."

It had been quite a week.

The center would open to the public by summer of 1966 at a dedication service where board member

Henry V. Scheirer would be the main speaker, the same man who was the main speaker at that dedication of the first dispensary twenty-eight years earlier.

"If anyone can find the wherewithal to finance the future of The Good Shepherd Home, it's Dr. Conrad Raker," Scheirer said. "So don't worry. The future is in good hands.

"To many people all over this land, The Good Shepherd Home is an opportunity to express love to a group who hunger for it."

And as Connie had predicted to the board earlier, organizations and agencies throughout Pennsylvania were now looking upon Good Shepherd as a dynamic growing institution for the care of the physically handicapped.

To carry the cause further, Connie sent letters and brochures about the center to every physician, member of the clergy and lawyer in the Lehigh Valley.

His letters to the doctors said the center was ready to welcome their referrals for rehabilitation. To the clergy, his text was just to alert them to the new services Good Shepherd was providing.

To the lawyers, he urged them where they saw the opportunity to suggest Good Shepherd for inclusion in their clients' wills. It was the renewal of a practice Papa instituted almost from the beginning of Good Shepherd.

And soon after the opening of this building, Connie was already dreaming aloud about another major project—a high-rise extended care facility for severely disabled individuals. That, however, would be a dozen years away.

The immediate need was a renovated North Wing of the main building as a hospital facility equipped to care for twenty-two bedridden or longtime rehabilitation patients. That would be ready by fall 1967.

Meanwhile, the opening of the rehabilitation center quickly set Good Shepherd off in a multitude of directions to further reclaim the battered and the broken.

Within months, it became the first extended care facility under Medicare in the area.

And in that first year also, the Home brought in Ray Crissey as administrative assistant in charge of the rehabilitation center. It took a good bit of persuasion by Connie to get Ray to accept.

Ray had worked in physical therapy for several years at the Reading, Pennsylvania, Rehabilitation Hospital, then went to Northeastern University for a master's in rehabilitation administration. And from there, he thought he was on his way to a job he had agreed to take in California.

But a friend had recommended Ray for Good Shepherd. Connie wrote him letters. Then, he phoned. "He was persistent," Ray says. "He wouldn't give up."

Ray came down from Boston to visit Good Shepherd and listen to Connie's plan for the rehabilitation center. "I went back to Boston," Ray recalls. "Connie phoned again and convinced my wife, and we decided to come."

And for Ray, a Seventh Day Adventist, he saw in this work at Good Shepherd the fulfilling of a yearning for a missionary role for his life.

And with the appointment in 1967 of Dr. Clifford H. Trexler, a noted Allentown surgeon, as chief of staff, what he was involved with was now called The Good Shepherd Rehabilitation Center and Hospital. His job was to guide more than 150 staff physicians and other professionals now serving the rehabilitation complex.

Sweet Charity proclaimed, "The demands placed upon The Good Shepherd Home are those of a modern medical complex."

Blue Cross signed a contract with Good Shepherd in 1968.

And Ray provided an update and evaluation in 1969 for the previous three years that might seem modest by today's achievements, but were extensive then:

The staff was 140 area physicians, three full-time physical therapists and two assistants, an occupational therapist and three assistants, sixteen registered nurses, twenty-six licensed practical nurses, three vocational counselors, a psychologist, social worker and limb maker.

From October 1965 to 1968, the rehabilitation center and hospital had served 125 inpatients and 285 outpatients, not including Good Shepherd's long-term residents.

There is a litany of services the center and hospital began providing. Colleges and universities started sending students for internships. So did nursing schools and regular hospitals.

The center and rehabilitation hospital fairly bristled with pride in 1971 when it became the third institution in Pennsylvania and twenty-ninth in the country certified by the Commission of Accreditation of Rehabilitation Facilities. It was the only one in the state certified in more than one area—physical restoration, vocational adjustment and sheltered employment.

It would be one of many distinctions to be bestowed upon the operation.

In the march toward developing the Conrad W. Raker Center for profoundly disabled permanent residents of Good Shepherd, and the new four-story rehabilitation hospital at the eastern end of the complex, both of them reaching completion during the administration of Dale Sandstrom, there is one relatively small item that should be included—a therapeutic pool.

It contains special lifts to lower litter patients directly into the water. The water is maintained at skin temperature for patient comfort and to receive a maximum therapeutic effect.

The floor of the pool is tiered, resulting in water depths ranging from three to five feet. And there are rails at each level to hold onto.

It was closed in the early months of this eightieth anniversary year because of the construction of the hospital addition. Ray Crissey says it's the one service people ask the most about.

It was built in the mid-1970s largely with money from Hal Dornsife, a steel mill owner from California, to honor his mother, Jennie Dornsife, of Nashville, Tennessee.

Ray wrote an article in the early 1970s about the hospital's needs. In response came a letter from Hal Dornsife about wanting to do something. At Connie's behest, Ray sent back a list of equipment.

Ray recalls, "This fellow wrote back and said that I misunderstood, that he wanted to make a major contribution."

Connie remembers that he had a "Dear Cousin" exchange of letters with Dornsife—making note that his grandmother Raker had been a Dornsife. And he says it turned out that this California Dornsife was some type of second cousin.

Connie says the upshot was that Dornsife contributed $40,000 toward the $75,000 cost of the pool.

Connie Raker undoubtedly didn't realize he was building his own monument with the construction of the four-story resident facility for severely handicapped people at the northwest corner of Sixth and St. John. That was virtually the spot where his parents had taken in the first crippled child.

The project was announced in early 1978 by Connie with a model of the structure. It was needed because Good Shepherd had a waiting list of 330. Another factor was increased state and federal requirements on the older buildings.

Half the expected $4 million cost was already on hand from friends and from some squirreled away by the board of trustees. Pennsylvania Power & Light Co. president Robert K. Campbell was heading the campaign committee to raise the remaining $2 million.

The building would provide beds for almost a hundred profoundly disabled people (representing an increase of a third) with balconies for the residents' privacy, comfort and enjoyment.

There would also be physical therapy and occupational therapy departments and a chapel.

But above all, Connie stressed, it would be designed to provide a home-like atmosphere for the residents.

Amid that first year of planning for this project, the Rev. Dale E. Sandstrom, a man Connie personally selected, began as assistant administrator for what was now referred to in *Sweet Charity* as The Good Shepherd Home and Rehabilitation Hospital.

And if Dale was someone Connie wanted, that alone was recommendation enough for most people.

Ground was broken May 6, 1979, with Connie Raker and his only surviving sister, Roberta (Raker) Hudders, holding the shovel together at a cross marked on the ground to turn the first spadeful of earth . . . the Roberta who had been part of the band trips in the early 1920s, who had helped supervise the girls for their camping experiences along the Little Lehigh in that same era, who had taught at the Home's school and who had directed some of the Anniversary Day pageants in those early years.

By then, the fund drive for the building was over the top. And what a blessing that was. The final cost had risen to $5 million. This project would be financed entirely by private gifts.

Connie Raker stepped aside as administrator on March 26, 1980, and Dale Sandstrom took over on that day.

It was in the aftermath of that changeover of leadership that Dale and the rest of the board decided to name the new building the Conrad W. Raker Center. It was dedicated that August 17 as "an institution of love and of the church fulfilling its purpose of witnessing to the community."

It was a fitting tribute to the man who presented the cause for forty-three years.

And in 1982, there was a smiling Dale Sandstrom on the cover of *Sweet Charity*, pointing to a spot at Fifth and St. John for a three-story rehabilitation hospital addition—right up against the rehabilitation center, the building with the Twenty-third Psalm.

It would enable Good Shepherd to add thirty-four beds to its existing twenty-six-bed hospital. All sixty beds were to be located in the addition.

Outpatients were coming in every day by the dozens for therapy. This addition would provide more quarters for those people who should be living in the hospital for the month or two it may take to restore them— people, for instance, like those with severe head injuries from accidents in small cars.

The emergency room crews of acute care hospitals were saving more of these people. But once a life has been saved, then rehabilitation is needed to enable these trauma patients to recover to their full potential and return to independence.

The project would require $3 million.

Even before this project was finished, Dale was saying, "We have one of the finest and most comprehensive rehabilitation centers throughout the country."

Those words came in 1983, the seventy-fifth anniversary of Good Shepherd. "Good Shepherd has a great legacy," he said. "She also has a great mandate to continue in the strong tradition of loving service in the next seventy-five years."

Just like Papa, just like Connie, Dale was looking at Good Shepherd beyond his own lifetime.

The dedication that July 31 was one of the high points on the seventy-fifth anniversary observance.

Lutheran Bishop Wilson E. Touhsaent told the dedication audience of 700 that "this institution has always recognized the source of all healing and help is in the Creator, God and Jesus Christ incarnate. We don't do it. He does it . . . through us, through the medical skills, through tremendous advances that have been made in all kinds of therapy to help people be restored to the maximum health of which they are capable."

August 2, the staff and patients moved in. And the place has been an increasingly thriving proposition ever since.

A back-page item in the January-February 1984 *Sweet Charity* gave an indication of the growth: "The opening of the rehabilitation hospital has meant an increase in staff at Good Shepherd. Since May, 104 full and part-time employees have joined the Good Shepherd family."

The spring of 1985 alone saw four new programs launched at the rehabilitation hospital:

—Cardiopulmonary rehabilitation for those with heart and lung problems where the patient's physician believes the individual would not benefit enough from a standard outpatient exercise program.

—Chronic pain management to help those with persistent pain and their families by learning how to cope with that pain.

—Spinal cord injury program with a goal to have each patient leave functioning as independently as possible.

—Head trauma program to guide patient and family through acceptance and adjustment to whatever disabilities result.

Those terms have a certain formality to them, correct as they are to the professionals who carry them out.

But there are still the glorious warm stories of what happens to people at Good Shepherd, just as there always have been.

In 1986, Martha Larson Martin of East Stroudsburg wrote to the staff about her sister Marie:

"Marie arrived at Good Shepherd after thirty-two days at Pocono Hospital. She was paralyzed on her left side. On the eleventh day at Good Shepherd Rehabilitation Hospital, she was discharged, able to walk without a cane or walker and with no noticeable limp.

"Marie had come to live with me right after my husband's death in 1977. Thus, with your help, Pocono's help and the Lord's, we had nine years of happy companionship until her death in February 1986.

"When I filled in the admission questionnaire for Marie at Good Shepherd, I wrote that my goal for her at your hospital was that she would become well enough to move about easily in a wheelchair so that I could bring her home to take care of her.

"Instead, she came home walking!"

Ray Crissey, the rehab hospital director, says, "Our program is intense. We have one of the shortest lengths of stay of any rehabilitation hospital in the country." The average stay is twenty-five days.

And in a mid-morning tour of the patient rooms, nobody's there. "They have to get up and get moving," Ray explains.

Families of patients who at first were in acute care hospitals were used to visiting their loved ones for weeks in the rooms. The patients are transferred to Good Shepherd. Ray says, "The families come in the next day to see them and they're not in their rooms. They're in therapy."

The place was outgrown almost from the time it opened. So here in this eightieth anniversary year, Good Shepherd is completing a fourth floor on the hospital for patients recuperating from head injuries.

The goal was nearly $3.7 million for a "Challenge for Hope and Healing"—to include the hospital expansion.

One phase of this was $1 million for a newly created endowment fund. Gifts for that nearly doubled the goal with $1.8 million by spring 1988.

The campaign called for nearly $2.7 million for that neurological care unit, space for therapeutic recreation, a hospital chapel and some related services. The goal for that phase was being approached in the eightieth anniversary year.

The result was total giving in the campaign of almost $5 million by June 1988.

In the beginning of Good Shepherd, Papa Raker often talked of how the Home took in infants only hours old and also welcomed Aunt Polly Nauman at age 106.

Here in this eightieth anniversary year, Good Shepherd Rehabilitation Hospital's many services range from a neonatal program to monitor the progress of premature infants to aiding those late in life who have endured amputations and strokes.

Ray Crissey says the joy of this work is the sense of inner satisfaction that you have contributed something worthwhile every day.

He says there's no better feeling than to be uptown and run into former patients. "They stop you. They want to introduce their whole family to you. They say they never would have made it if it hadn't been for Good Shepherd.

"They're so excited. They make you feel as if you had done it all by yourself." ❖

When I need to be cheered, I come to The Good Shepherd Home, where bodies are comforted and spirits lifted.

Rev. Charles J. Harris
Sweet Charity
March-May 1947

There is a multitude of stories from the later decades of Good Shepherd that tell every bit as much what a caring place it is as do those from the early years.

And scattered amid them are tales of heartache and sorrow that could be devastating to the human spirit.

Connie Raker has said that Good Shepherd is a Protestant Boys Town. It garners the support of devout believers of many faiths beyond the borders of its Lutheran origins, including many Catholics and Jews.

But it is not the story of the happy-go-lucky Papa Raker, the always-jolly Connie Raker or Dale Sandstrom as the smiling Scandinavian.

These are people who have been tested by devastation.

Papa felt fulfillment in placing a young girl in a loving family. But he was hit by a touch of sadness because the natural mother finally showed up after eleven years to ask about her.

Tucked away in one of Connie's reports to the board in the 1950s are the details about the deeply depressed spastic resident who came into his own room, locked his door, walked right by his spastic roommate who could not get off his bed, opened a window and plunged to his death.

Connie, who had agonized over that troubled soul, had to get up the next day to face the world around him. So did that spastic roommate, Jim Kerrigan. Connie has inspired so many with his quiet leadership. Jim has given so many of us joy and friendship over the years just by waving from his wheelchair at Sixth and St. John. Dare we ask more courage than that of either one?

Did you catch the brief item in a 1985 *Sweet Charity* about the Raker Center resident whose family has visited him only twice in fifty-five years? Papa lived through some of that, so did Connie and now so does Dale.

Then, there's Billy Anderson. He had that pioneering arm operated by carbon dioxide until he decided he could manage better with paint brushes and such by just holding them between his shoulder and his chin. He was a whiz at painting signs for the State Highways Department with a paintbrush under his chin.

He got to Washington to pose with some of the top leadership of the U.S. Senate. If there were stars at Good Shepherd, surely he was one. And then a fire that he could not escape brought an end to his life in his early 20s.

God, what pain to the Good Shepherd people who nurtured Billy as he grew and who helped him to go out on his own.

*   *   *

But Good Shepherd is essentially a song of triumph amid those heartaches. Maybe in part it's because the battered and broken bodies that make their way to Good Shepherd and the people who care for them help others beyond their doors.

Papa, for all his fighting with synod leaders, took two weeks off in 1912 to go out and work in a synod $500,000 campaign in behalf of Muhlenberg College and Mt. Airy Seminary.

"The superintendent of Good Shepherd has his hands full trying to make ends meet at the Home," *Sweet Charity* said. "We, however, want the synod plan to succeed. The members of the board of the Home have consented that the superintendent spend two weeks collecting for the fund as Good Shepherd's contribution to the cause."

Sweet Charity devoted a whole page to the Allentown YMCA campaign of 1915.

And at Christmas 1919, kind friends and organizations had donated so liberally that the Home was supplied with everything needed. So the Home children shared their bounty with other poor children in the neighborhood who had little or nothing.

The Home was overwhelmed in August 1922 when the Elks of Bethlehem arrived with 1,700 boxes each containing a ham and cheese sandwich, a peach and a pickle.

"We ate sandwiches until we almost turned into sandwiches," Papa reported. "We took a load to the farms. We called the Day Nursery and gave them a liberal supply. We offered a box to all who passed the Home and looked hungry.

"We took a load around the Twelfth Ward and gave freely to the children. Still, there was danger that some might spoil.

"We took a load on the auto to Wire Street. Here, the children completely surrounded the machine and stopped all traffic. We supplied all but five. Those five we brought to the Home on the auto and gave them two boxes each.

"It is not often that an orphanage is compelled to say: 'Stop! It is enough. ' "

And when the Depression came and the Home had hardly enough for itself, there were hungry unemployed men at the door—sometimes as many as fifty in a single day—who were given a meal.

How do you measure in human achievement the sweet charity of Good Shepherd taking in widows and abandoned women with small children in those early decades . . . the women to be given a job plus shelter and food to be able to provide for their little ones.

When the Lowman Home for Epileptics at White Rock, South Carolina, was in financial trouble in the 1930s, Good Shepherd sent $100 and put an appeal in *Sweet Charity* to help. What Good Shepherd did spread throughout the South. People there said that if a place like Good Shepherd could help, surely they could, too.

When the National Lutheran Council reported 250 refugees who were Lutherans in New York at the onset of World War II, Good Shepherd took a doctor, his wife and three children until they could become fully established in America. And Good Shepherd sent a check to the National Lutheran Council as well to help it with its work.

There was also the fact that the kids of the neighborhood could come in and take meals with their friends who lived at the Home. A basketball court on the grounds for years served the youngsters of the neighborhood as much as those who were Home children. And by the hundreds, children of the ward attended free movies that Good Shepherd showed.

The Home began with Papa Raker sending every child he could up St. John Street to the Jefferson School for his basic education. Some had to be hauled there by coaster wagon.

Here, as this eightieth anniversary unfolds, Raker Center residents are still involved with Jefferson School—serving as teacher's aides to help pupils with their studies.

That, too, has come back in special blessings. In 1987, Jefferson School students, teachers and friends donated $605 toward a new wheelchair for Scott Sandler, one of their aides from Good Shepherd.

And here in this anniversary year, Patricia Weaver, Jefferson's immediate past principal, has been cited by the Pennsylvania State Education Association for her work in fostering the teacher's aides program of Raker Center people. Allentown Education Association nominated Weaver for the award.

An item in the March-April 1983 *Sweet Charity* noted that Good Shepherd residents, feeling they have the necessities of life while many others do not, contributed part of their Sunday chapel offering during the previous six months to help pay the heating bills of a needy family in Bethlehem, purchase baby food for the poor and go toward medicine for a needy person.

When the rehabilitation hospital opened in 1983, new X-ray equipment was installed because the old unit was too small. That old unit was donated to Curran Lutheran Hospital in Monrovia, Liberia, with the assistance of the Division of World Mission and Ecumenism of the Lutheran Church in America.

Good Shepherd employees have donated money for the World Hunger Appeal. So has the chapel council— with most of that coming from Sunday offerings of Raker Center residents from the $25 a month allowance they receive from their Social Security.

And the often-serenaded residents at Raker Center go out on their wheelchairs to serenade their St. John Street neighbors with carols at Christmas.

The "Hands Across America" chain did not wind its way through Allentown in 1986. But another special chain linked hands at Good Shepherd one day that spring.

They called the event "Hands around Good Shepherd." Residents, patients, clients, staff and volunteers clasped hands around the main campus to express concern for the hungry. Everyone sang "Hands Across America" and "We Are the World." Those joining the line donated money or canned food for the Lehigh Valley Food Bank.

* * *

There has been a rather illustrious list of famous people who have visited the Home over the years. It seems almost expected that Dale Sandstrom secures some sports star to be among the speakers each fall when Good Shepherd inducts someone into its Handicapped Hall of Fame, what with his background in college and professional football.

Pennsylvania Governor Gifford Pinchot, the

conservationist from the Poconos, visited the Home sometime in late 1925. But it got only a line mention in *Sweet Charity*, and that wasn't Papa's usual style when there was mileage to be gotten for the Home for any event.

Jack Dempsey, the heavyweight boxing champion, visited Good Shepherd while he was in Allentown in January 1933 for a one-week engagement. The Home band performed for him. The fact that some band members were crippled and one without arms especially caught Dempsey's attention.

In the sun parlor, Dempsey gave what was described as an excellent Sunday school speech. He advised the boys to take good care of their bodies and not to smoke, at least not until they were twenty-one.

Of all the institutions he had visited, Good Shepherd made the deepest impression. "There's a case where people are really doing some good out in the world. They surely are."

And years later, when Jersey Joe Walcott, another heavyweight boxing champion, stopped at Good Shepherd for the first time, Mama Raker quickly let him know she had already shaken hands with Dempsey.

When the Army-Navy game was played in 1937, $100 of the game proceeds went to The Good Shepherd Home. The academies had a policy of donating money to a charity that each player designated. And for Cadet Charles R. Meyer of Allentown, his selection was Good Shepherd.

That cadet was later known as Gen. Charles R. "Monk" Meyer, just in this eightieth anniversary year feted at a testimonial dinner at the Grand Ballroom of the Waldorf-Astoria in New York City. The event was for an award as a "great American" from the National Football Foundation and Hall of Fame.

It was rather appropriate that the Rev. Walter Eastwood of Allentown's First Presbyterian Church would be writing an extended message in 1946 in the pages of *Sweet Charity*—perhaps the first non-Lutheran member of the clergy to be writing there, rather than being written about.

Thousands of people with many religious backgrounds had given to Good Shepherd over those first forty years. But First Presbyterian, with two of its members as guests at the Home, had been the first congregation of any denomination to include Good Shepherd in its annual budget.

Cowboy actors Roy Rogers and his wife, Dale Evans, stopped at the Home during a 1959 appearance at the Allentown Fair to greet the youngsters and pose for pictures with them in the parlor of the main building. And then they visited in the rooms with those who couldn't be moved into the parlor.

In 1962, they came back again during fair week for a visit in mid-week. And one morning of that week, Connie was among a small party invited to join Roy Rogers for some skeet shooting at a local rod and gun club. Connie calls it "divine intervention" that he beat the Hollywood cowboy in the skeet competition.

More important, when he learned Roy Rogers had no place in mind for worship the coming Sunday, Connie invited him to join the Good Shepherd community in the chapel. Both Roy and Dale showed up unannounced that Sunday for worship with the residents. And like the earlier time, they went around the rooms afterward to greet those residents confined to their beds.

Other celebrities, like Lawrence Welk and Johnny Cash, included Good Shepherd amid their Allentown Fair appearances.

Mrs. Muriel Humphrey stopped by in 1972 to see the rehabilitation facilities. And later that year, so did Mrs. Elliot L. Richardson and Mrs. Donald Rumsfeld—to tour the workshop.

And, of course, over the years, leaders of the Lutheran Church have made pilgrimages to Good Shepherd, often as speakers at anniversary day programs.

And in the mail, President William Howard Taft was among those sending greetings to Aunt Polly Nauman upon her 107th birthday on Sept. 11, 1912.

President John F. Kennedy sent a letter in 1962 to guest Billy Luppold who used his toes to sketch. "I want to extend my heartiest congratulations on your ability to draw, as well as write and type, under such tremendous handicaps," he wrote.

And Sharon Pasquinelli, a blind resident, met Lady Bird Johnson when the president's wife made an appearance at Allentown's Center Square in 1964.

"I was chosen to give the flowers. I was about seventeen or eighteen. The security men had to open the flowers and check them before I was to give them to her."

Not only did Mrs. Johnson take time then to talk with Sharon, the first lady afterward sent her a special delivery letter, praising her courage for managing with both blindness and other disabilities that have kept her in a wheelchair.

* * *

Just to give some indication of what a bustling place the rehabilitation program has become, a woman by the name of Diane Counterman was admitted in early 1987 for several weeks in the aftermath of a car accident. She came and went without anyone learning who she really was.

She was a granddaughter of Viola Hunt, the first child admitted to Good Shepherd. ❖

I believe the greatest frustration for all handicapped persons is that an hour is not a full sixty minutes.

Betty Ruth Pumphrey
Sweet Charity
July-August 1964

Betty Ruth Pumphrey says she didn't know Conrad Raker's name when she wrote in 1956 to inquire about being admitted to The Good Shepherd Home. She simply addressed the envelope: "Superintendent, Good Shepherd Home, Allentown, Pa."

It arrived.

And back came a copy of *Sweet Charity* and *The Open Door,* a pamphlet of pictures and message of the Home's history. "I fell in love with the place," Betty Ruth says.

She arrived June 14, 1963, a young woman with cerebral palsy and a lot of talent, and has been at the Home ever since. She could still walk then. She's in a wheelchair now. She is a Good Shepherd institution, known for her writing, probably the only wheelchair resident of Raker Center who has been to the Louvre and to come away to write a poem about it.

She's among a cross-section of people who have been involved with Good Shepherd—some only briefly, others like Betty Ruth for much of their lives—who were interviewed for this book.

Some had their words woven into stories in other chapters. Some are here on these pages.

If there's a general theme running through what they have to say, it is that they have received more in return from Good Shepherd than anything they have given.

Betty Ruth's father was a professor and dean of engineering at Auburn University. And she makes a special point to note that she is a teacher's aide at Jefferson Elementary just up the street from Good Shepherd.

"I love it, first and second grade, Tuesdays and Thursdays," she says.

She enjoys the times when Connie Raker has a meal with Raker Center residents. "Even though he's semi-retired, he comes over to eat, usually at noon. It's a chance to visit with him."

* * *

John Shepherd of Emmaus, born in 1916, was found on the doorstep of Good Shepherd when he was about three months old. Dr. Wackernagel baptized him. He says he has two birthdays, the day he was born and the day he was found at the Home.

He was one of the normals. For nine years, he took care of Teddy, a dog the boys had in the Home. "Teddy always slept on my bed at night." As John grew up in the Home, one of his jobs was to clean, dress and undress a helpless boy every day.

Mama Raker was one of the greatest, John says. "She took care of us boys when we were real young. She had a sense of humor, very intelligent, one of the shrewdest.

"When she'd tell you something, you had to do it. There was never no second time to tell you, never.

"Papa was away quite often, trying to get finances from the Lutheran people. She ran the place until she got into her 60s."

John retired in 1974 after thirty-three years as a production worker with Mack Trucks. He has a wife and four children.

* * *

Neighbor Randolph Kulp, who has lived all his six decades at the southwest corner of 6th and St. John streets, is a son of a trolley car driver.

He recalls that back when he was a kid, Papa Raker would arrange to have the Good Shepherd children admitted to a movie uptown. Then, he'd phone the Lehigh Valley Transit Co. to get it to bring a trolley out—for free—to transport the youngsters to the movie.

Randy would go along as did some other neighbor children. "The motormen knew me because of my dad. They'd kid me, saying: 'Hey, you're not a Good Shepherd Home boy.' I went to three of those movies that way."

And he recalls the armless Martin Revelette, a youngster with mischief in his heart, who had his own personal fund-raising methods. Martin and two of his pals with a dog would go uptown. "People would be reaching in their pockets for money to give them."

It was because of stunts like that that Papa Raker repeatedly admonished *Sweet Charity* readers to give their contributions directly to the Home, not to the children individually. Too much money in young hands could make for problems.

* * *

She was Susan Endres of Rutherford, New Jersey, a senior at Muhlenberg College in the spring of 1976 and an intern social worker at Good Shepherd since the previous fall.

There had been a hundred young men and women from various universities and colleges the year before who benefited from training at Good Shepherd in their work to become rehabilitation professionals. Besides Muhlenberg, they had been from schools like Cedar Crest, Lafayette, Kutztown and Moravian.

What set Susan apart was that she was blind since birth.

"Good Shepherd's all I expected it to be and more," Susan said near the end of her internship. "The staff really cares and goes out of its way to help both patients and guests. A true spirit of love and dedication pervades everything that goes on."

In this eightieth anniversary year, she is Susan
Wojtecki of Orange, New Jersey, married and the
mother of a two-year-old son. She has a master's
degree in social work from the State University at
Albany, New York.

Good Shepherd was a good kind of beginning
experience, she says. "It enabled me to integrate the
things I was learning in the classroom." She still
remembers that Mary Ellen Place was her supervisor.

It was a generally happy experience. "You were
working with families to prepare them so the patients
could leave."

While at graduate school, Susan served in a nursing
facility where the patients were terminally ill. And she
has since been on the staff of an agency counseling
victims of domestic violence.

None of these later experiences has had the positive
quality that came in serving at Good Shepherd, Susan
says.

*   *   *

Roberta (Raker) Hudders, Connie's lone surviving
sibling, has great trouble with her speech because of a
stroke. She labors mightily to get out even short
stories to be a part of this book. But her eyes tell a
yearning to share what she remembers.

For a number of years, she says she was barred from
the band trips because she couldn't play a musical
instrument. Finally, she was allowed to go along.

She picked potatoes on the Good Shepherd farms
like all the other kids. "I had to," she says.

Her higher education had started at Marion Junior
College in Virginia. But she left there after being
accused of wearing rouge, when what she had was
simply a rosy-cheeked face.

She transferred to Wittenberg in Ohio, another
Lutheran school, and was an outstanding student. But
for a long period, she didn't write home.

This prompted Papa to write the school officials: "Is
daughter Roberta safe?"

The school responded: "Daughter Roberta is safe."

Safe, surely, but when she came home the next time, she had bobbed hair and was promptly labeled one of the "bobbed-hair bandits."

Even after her marriage in 1932, she taught at Good Shepherd and directed its pageants.

*   *   *

Catherine "Kitty" Smicker of Allentown is a volunteer who got involved with Good Shepherd through Red Cross twenty years ago and has been involved ever since.

She phoned the Red Cross asking where she could do volunteer work. And shortly after that, she met some of the Good Shepherd youngsters at the Frick Boat Club on the Lehigh River. Her husband, John, was club president, and each year the club gave Good Shepherd youngsters a boat ride as their rental for use of Adams Island as a headquarters.

Afterward, the club had a picnic for the visitors. Kitty says once she met those kids from Good Shepherd, she concluded, "I think I'd like to work over there."

Her work is not just for one or two. "I do for all," she says.

"I'm at the hospital every Friday. They're new faces, a great bunch. At Raker Center, it's a lot of letter writing, pushing them where they have to go, feeding them."

She was particularly attached to the old folks, who were part of Good Shepherd until about ten years ago.

"I'm Ukrainian. My mom died in childbirth and left six little ones. I didn't know what it was to have a mom. I just took to the older people. I just loved them.

"One thing kind of gets to me: When they pass on, that hurts.

"People sometimes ask me how could I work there. Well, I've had bad days, too, and they perked me up. They're a jolly bunch with always a thank you.

"And I can't say enough about Dr. Raker. He will never pass you up without a little pat, a hug, asking you how the family is.

"I feed at lunchtime at Raker Center. He'll come in. He'll have lunch with the residents. I think that's so nice.

"Every day, something is going on. Now, everyone gets therapy. So it's a busy place.

"It's like a big family. It's like caring for your own."

* * *

Marguerite "Tinker" Ruhf is an unabashed Connie Raker groupie. "I thought he was very cute when I worked there in the late 1940s. I still think he's cute."

It was in the immediate aftermath of World War II that Tinker married and came home to Allentown looking for a job. She worked in occupational therapy during 1947-49 at Good Shepherd and attracted enough attention to wind up on covers of *Sweet Charity* twice.

"The work paid $50 a month, and that paid the rent," she recalls. She and colleague Sally Collins had the task of training people to do something, to give them a feeling of self-respect.

"Physical therapy is basically exercise. We were moving arms and legs that should be moved. We used a lot of crafts. The end result was not what was made. The important thing was what happened to people."

This was an era when the local crippled children's society ran a day camp near Allentown's trout hatchery that some Good Shepherd youngsters attended. "When it came to going to day camp, we loaded them up in the body of an open truck. The kids loved it. But nobody would allow that today."

The kids who could stand and maintain their balance were allowed to go in the stream. Others were limited to a nearby pond. But they all got a chance to get their feet wet.

"George Goldfus wanted to stand. That was his goal. He couldn't walk, but he could stand," Tinker says.

And she also recalls Jeff Steinberg, a Philadelphia boy with no arms and only part of his legs. "Jeff was a pistol, aggressive. I guess when you're like that, you fight all the way.

"That guy on his little legs would chase the girls. He'd ride a coaster wagon, fly down the hill. At camp, he was a puppeteer. He was a clever, bright boy. He wanted to run everything."

For some reason, she remembers stewed celery tops. "It was the first time I ever had stewed celery tops. That was using up everything."

She says it was truly a home while she was there. "It was a good home, a loving home."

* * *

The applause went on and on in Grace Lutheran Church for James "Jimmy" Boyle when Good Shepherd honored him at an anniversary program in February 1988. This was a Home crowd showing its appreciation for a Home boy who has spent nearly all his sixty-five years tied to Good Shepherd.

He was a child when he was brought to the Home from Tamaqua.

"I never knew my father. My mother worked."

To Jimmy, like many other youngsters, Mama Raker was his mother. "She was a lovely person. She'd help us clear the meal tables. She'd make sure we'd say our prayers every night."

Papa was someone who was often out on the road, raising money for the Home. Jimmy says Papa had an old Dodge that he'd load up with eighteen kids and take them out to the farm.

The boys were in a dorm, fifteen on each side. "Oh, we had pillow fights! We had fun like other kids. When we'd get hungry at night, we'd put one of the smallest kids in the dumbwaiter and put him down to the pantry to get food.

"A lot of people say the grass is greener on the other side. But you couldn't ask for a nicer institution. I'm very proud and thankful to be a part of The Good Shepherd Home.

"You had all the opportunities you wanted to go through college and get your education. If I wanted to, I would have. I only went to the first year of high school."

Jimmy joined the Civilian Conservation Corps in 1938. He came back from that and then went into the Army. But even in those years, he felt he still had a home at Good Shepherd.

After the war, Jimmy worked for a time at Hess Brothers. "In 1950, Dr. Raker asked if I'd come and help at the Home, work on the grounds, chauffeur, drive the kids to school."

He recalls carrying Jeff Steinberg up and down the steps of a synagogue every week at Sixth and Tilghman Streets on the north side of town for his religious instruction. "And I took Billy Anderson all over."

At one time, Jimmy was overseer of most everything at Good Shepherd. His position in this eightieth anniversary year is materials manager.

Jimmy and his wife Ruth were married in the Good Shepherd chapel. Their children were baptized there. Ruth herself worked at the Home for thirty-five years. She died in 1982.

Jimmy has seen vast changes at Good Shepherd across his lifetime. "It has grown and grown. Yet, it still has love and compassion for everybody."

* * *

Evelyn Scheirer is a year older than The Good Shepherd Home, and for about the last sixty years she has been music teacher to generations of its residents. She is a graduate of Cedar Crest College.

She grew up in the neighborhood of St. Luke's Lutheran Church on the north side of town. As a youngster, she heard about Good Shepherd through Dr. Wackernagel, who was affiliated with her church. "He talked Good Shepherd," she says.

In 1925, the Rev. William Katz came to St. Luke's. He formed a Luther League, and one of its projects was to do something for someone else. Twice a year, Evelyn was involved in a St. Luke's program at Good Shepherd.

One of the residents, Harry Filer, was attending

Muhlenberg College. He was a singer of some note, Papa billing him as the Home's Caruso.

"Our pastor soon had Harry singing on our choir. He needed an accompanist, so I accompanied him for a couple years."

In the winter of 1927, Mama Raker asked her to teach piano to the youngsters. Evelyn had her own regular pupils and worked in those at Good Shepherd.

She thinks it was Mama that had everything to do with her hiring. Papa told her the board was not hiring that day at its meeting.

But Mama took her aside and asked her for all the information about the music lessons so she could present it to the board. "Then she called me and said the board approved.

"I played for all the pageants. For a while, I was coaching teenagers to play the organ for chapel services. They had talented youngsters. Then, one by one they left. Then, one got sick.

"I volunteered to play the chapel organ in 1949. I thought it would be for a few weeks. I was there until 1985."

She directed the Good Shepherd choir. "I was paid for one rehearsal a week. But I would practice with them every day."

She and Mama became close friends. "Mama Raker was the kindest woman I ever knew. When my mother died, she said, 'When you get lonely, you come to us. You know who your friends are.'

"I missed my mother and she sort of filled in. If she wanted to go somewhere, she'd ask me to take her."

Evelyn says she's had times of illness when Good Shepherd took care of her for a week, maybe longer. "And that was Mama Raker's doing," she says.

When Evelyn moved to 522 St. John Street in 1953, she could wave across the street to Mama in the Old Folks Building at the corner of Fifth and St. John.

Every day after lunch, Mama made the rounds of the old folks' quarters. "Just the thought she was at the door and gave them a friendly greeting meant a great deal to them." ❖

HERE WE GROW AGAIN

Headline
Sweet Charity
May-June 1986

When Dale Sandstrom was considering coming to Good Shepherd, Connie Raker put his hand on his shoulder and said, "I don't want you to look at Good Shepherd for what it is now. Look at it for what it can become."

And what a place Good Shepherd has become in what might be called Dale's Decade.

Or should it be places (plural)?

Because with satellite units in communities like Kutztown and South Whitehall Township, the rehabilitation hospital with all its ramifications is a sprawling network.

Because with satellite units and several thrift shops, Industrial Services and Vocational Services have people working all over the Lehigh Valley.

Because with individual units around the community, the independent living phase of Good Shepherd has physically challenged people—we don't say "handicapped" or "crippled" anymore—out making it on their own.

Because with Carl Odhner and his wheelchair armada called Operation Overcome, barriers of steps and other architectural protuberances that have denied access to the physically disabled are disappearing.

Who is this Swede with the dimples, this grandson

of immigrants, who is leading this revolution in the heart of the Pennsylvania Dutch country? "There are not too many oddballs like me around," Dale says.

He sounds like Papa Raker when he says his whole background, his entire personal makeup, has prepared him for his work at Good Shepherd.

Isn't that pretty much what Papa said, that virtually everything he did had prepared him for starting The Good Shepherd Home?

And here in this eightieth anniversary year, Dale is getting an honorary doctor of divinity from Muhlenberg—just like Connie before him and Papa before him.

Papa got his D.D. at Muhlenberg's 1920 commencement, where Mabel Knecht of Allentown became the first woman to receive a diploma from the school. He said his honorary degree was actually the church giving full recognition to the Home. With Dale, that makes the recognition three-fold.

Each, however, has his own trademark . . . Papa with that delightfully stuffy picture of him, Mama and the three others of the founding board . . . Connie at the open door of the administration building, welcoming people to Good Shepherd . . . and Dale in shirtsleeves, holding Erin Santa, a child in the day school program.

Dale began life in North Dakota and was raised in Montana. He was an Evangelical Lutheran, a Norwegian Lutheran. It was a dedicated pastor and a layman, a beekeeper, in Montana who made such a deep impression on him that led him into the ministry.

He says he felt a strong desire to demonstrate the faith of the church. "The greatest witness of Good Shepherd is to witness God's love in the world," Dale says.

He was a football star at quarterback at Concordia College at Moorhead, Minnesota. In 1987, the school inducted him into its Athletic Hall of Fame for his athletic accomplishments and his "great service on behalf of handicapped people nationwide."

He was a twelfth-round draft choice of the Chicago Cardinals in 1954, a professional football team in the

National Football League, and played a year.

"In college, everybody thought I was going to go into coaching. People said: Why don't you make something of yourself? Go into coaching or something. What made you do a fool thing like going into the ministry?"

At Concordia, he was a senior when he met Lillian Gustavsen, a sophomore who came from a close-knit Norwegian community on Staten Island, New York. She was a member of what was then an American Lutheran congregation that had a pastor who wanted the young people to go west to a church college— either St. Olaf's or Concordia.

Lillian had to quit school after that sophomore year and return home to Staten Island because her father was ill. But she came home with an engagement ring from Dale.

She worked a year in Manhattan, then went west again to marry Dale while he was in his second year at Luther Theological Seminary in St. Paul. She worked in the church headquarters in Minneapolis. It was her income that put him through seminary.

She would delay the completion of her own undergraduate education until the early 1980s when she got a degree in library science with a minor in art from Kutztown University. And she would serve as a volunteer for story hour with the children at Good Shepherd's day school nursery. "I'm a librarian," she explains.

Meanwhile, there would be three Sandstrom children, Peter, now an electrical engineer in New Hampshire; Kari, a nurse at Pocono Hospital and wife of Attorney David Kutnik, and Marcus, assistant to the vice president for administration at Good Shepherd.

At this eightieth anniversary, Marcus has served at Good Shepherd four years. "I feel like part of a family here," he says. "There are a lot of good people."

A relative planted the seed in Dale's mind that he should go into hospital administration.

And when he was in parishes for a dozen years in Montana, Minnesota and then New York, that idea kept gnawing away at him. There were hundreds of vacancies in Lutheran parishes. But Dale yearned to do something more.

In Minnesota, there was a young man in his congregation in Elmore, who had been injured in a diving accident. Dale helped him almost every day for five years in his work on the parallel bars. One of his last visits of the day was to stop at this young man's home. And he shared the joy of this man's recovery. "I didn't realize then I'd be moving into rehabilitation."

Dale got his master's in business administration on Staten Island at Wagner College, then served a year's internship at Nyack Hospital, an acute care facility in New York State. He worked his way up to assistant vice president for administration in six years at that hospital before he left to come to Good Shepherd.

A search team out of Chicago located Dale for Good Shepherd. Connie Raker really didn't know him. But Dale says there were vibrations when they met.

Connie Raker had told the board that the job of running Good Shepherd was rapidly becoming more complicated. What was needed was someone with hospital administration experience—if possible, a Lutheran minister with that experience.

The board minutes of July 1978 tersely note that Connie informed the trustees they "would hopefully soon meet with a clergyman administrator of a hospital who has all the credentials both personal and professional for assistant administrator."

There were three finalists. The board met at the Livingston Club in Allentown to make its choice. The trustees asked Connie: Who do you want?

His choice was Dale.

And that October, with Dale in the job a month, the board minutes noted, "He has been taking hold of his work very well. His managerial skills were beginning to show."

Dale sees his immediate job as planning Good Shepherd for the next ten to twenty years. "We're in good shape financially. We're not big as business goes."

He says that when he came, no program was solvent. All were dependent in various degrees upon gifts from outside. Some, like Raker Center and

Vocational Services, have to be subsidized. "We still have to depend on the public."

But the rehabilitation hospital is self-supporting as well as being one of the most comprehensive in the country. And Good Shepherd is trying to develop a strong endowment plan.

Dale centers his comments upon the word wholistic. This dimension has caused such rapid growth and expansion. "I try to look at things from the standpoint of wholistic. Not parts of bodies, arms and legs, but the whole person—physically, mentally, socially, spiritually.

"The church has asked us to be responsible for a social ministry. We have wholistic counseling for families that are in disarray, a drug and alcohol program in counseling, an employee assistance program for those with social, economic and drug problems.

"We have to give a sense of dignity about self, a sense that your contributions are worth something to the world, that motivated you can do almost anything.

"That is paramount for Good Shepherd. Everybody has to latch onto that."

Dale says his work is demanding, exciting. "I love it."

And he finds that the people in the area are great— even though most of us aren't Swedish. But then his wife Lillian isn't either. Dale laughs when he says it took a bit of doing for his Norwegian mother-in-law to get over the fact that Lillian married a Swede.

No, he says, he has not been turned primarily into a fund-raiser. "Not yet."

He tries to get out to talk with the residents and patients. But he says there is never enough time to do that as often as he'd like, even with much of the daily business in the hands of senior vice presidents.

He sees among the achievements of his years at Good Shepherd "the expansion of the rehabilitation hospital with an excellence in programs which we didn't have before. The head injury program is second to none . . . spinal cord . . . chronic pain program . . . a strong industrial medicine program.

"We've been able to attract excellence in the medical staff. We raised the quality of our medical staff."

His biggest heartache is trying to put in motion an independent living program. "We've handicapped our people by trying to do everything for them."

The aim is to get them to do more on their own than ever before. He estimates that 20 percent of the 135 residents of Raker Center have the ability to do that.

But then the government inflicts financial "disincentives" upon those profoundly handicapped people who try to work their way toward independence. If they make too much money, and a very little bit is too much, then the government cuts back on their Social Security and other benefits.

Both Dale and rehabilitation hospital director Ray Crissey talk of developing what they label Good Shepherd Village.

It would be training for independent living with development of vocational skills thrown in where needed.

"This would be a village concept where the residents would have apartments to live on their own with a caretaker to look in on them. That's my dream. The ultimate goal would be independence," Dale says.

He sees it in the next five or ten years. These would be small groups in communal living. He says the federal government no longer finances projects involving large numbers in such groups.

Dale envisions a network of homes across the Lehigh Valley to house the disabled from where they can launch out into the community. "And we still may have some kind of core center around here at Good Shepherd."

The goal is for the disabled to be their own persons.

Dale is also toying with the idea of a national television program to expound the message of the disabled.

What marvelous things computers have done to put the physically challenged, the handicapped, on an achievement plane with those of us who are able-bodied. What one finger can do in punching keys!

Dale says everyone involved in Good Shepherd

together is helping the Home in its mission.

He has worked to develop a strong partnership with the churches in the area. For instance, since 1982, church councils from ninety congregations in the Lehigh Valley have been invited in for a meal and a tour of Good Shepherd. It began with Lutheran congregations and expanded to those of other faiths. Subsequent letters in *Sweet Charity* indicate this has been warmly received.

In initiating the invitations, Dale announced that the ministry of Good Shepherd needs to be shared jointly in a partnership fashion with the congregations and Good Shepherd as an agency of the Lutheran Church.

"God's message of love is not only expressed through the congregational life, but also through social action," Dale said at the outset.

What the Home learned was that many church council members had never visited Good Shepherd before.

This project is a somewhat expanded version of what Papa Raker used to do in having the seniors from Mt. Airy and Gettysburg Lutheran seminaries in for a chicken dinner and a tour. Papa reasoned they would soon be pastors of area churches who would be kindly disposed to help Good Shepherd.

For the seventy-fifth anniversary year, Connie Raker put together some reflections for *Sweet Charity* readers. He closed with these thoughts:

"We have spoken of the past. We have spoken briefly of the present. But what really is Good Shepherd?

"It is a group of modern, dedicated, well-trained men and women who are following the Lord's injunction— 'As much as ye have done it unto these, my brethren, ye have done it unto me.'

"The staff of Good Shepherd is, in essence, Good Shepherd. They daily breathe the breath of life into its on-going program. We can't sing their praise too highly.

"The rehabilitation team is performing modern twentieth-century New Testament miracles everyday.

"But what of the future?

"The future is in good hands.

"Rev. Dale Sandstrom, with a background in hospital administration, has thrown himself wholeheartedly into the cause of the handicapped. Under Dale's guidance, God will continue to bless Good Shepherd."

More people than ever need Good Shepherd's help.

With all the advances in medical technology, more and more people are surviving accidents and injuries that would have killed them a few years ago.

Surviving for what?

"Well, rehabilitation is what will make the difference in the quality of their lives," Dale responds to his own question. Rehabilitation may make the difference between being ambulatory or not, developing maximum independence or not, enjoying leisure time or being bored into depression.

To the vast Good Shepherd congregation, he says:

"We need your help so we can help the residents of Raker Center transcend the limitations of their physical disabilities and live the fullest life possible.

"We need your help so that people with physical, mental and emotional disabilities can learn to earn their own living and glory in the dignity of a job well done at the end of each work day."

Dale says that as Good Shepherd grows bigger, those running it must develop systems for working together.

"Something has changed, but nothing has changed. We're still a caring institution. We have the same caring and loving, the same sense of family. We know that all individuals have the right to the opportunity to be all they can be.

"We've all been called to do great things. Our people feel great inside because they've helped someone reach for a star.

"You can really move the world here at Good Shepherd." ❖

We have all been the mission of The Good Shepherd Home:

. . . those with tortured bodies whose lifetime will be spent essentially within its confines . . .

. . . those wayfarers injured along life's path who are there to spend a few weeks to be wooed or lovingly bullied into restoration or, at least, taught the lessons of daily survival . . .

. . . those who come and go in jobs the Home has provided in sheltered settings or, once growing ability is shown, in work out in the world with so-called normals . . .

. . . those who came by one day on a tour and just couldn't help coming back to volunteer . . .

. . . those who heard Papa Raker or Connie Raker or Dale Sandstrom speak and just felt they had to dig down in their pockets to aid the cause . . .

. . . those workers, employees, staff, the titles be damned, from top to bottom who have sent their spirit out across the land in just how they have treated those within their care and how they shared their concerns with the families . . .

. . . those who read *Sweet Charity* from distant miles and offered prayers . . .

. . . those now gone who struggled to create what those after have expanded and refined . . .

. . . and this one chosen writer, blessed beyond comprehension by having been asked to put this joyous, crazy, loving history together.

Good Shepherd has gotten to us all. It has stolen our hearts, just as Papa said it would. It has held us in its loving arms and we don't want to get away.

The guest speaker on Anniversary Day back in 1911 told the assemblage: "You are here laying the foundations of an institution that may stand for 500 or 1,000 years."

What glory to have been even a small part of it. ❖

BOARD MEMBERS

Evelyn Allen	1987 -
Wilson Arbogast	1915 - 1924
Robert Aten	1947 - 1947
Rev. Fred S. Blank	1959 - 1964
Dr. George S. Boyer	1981 -
Jerome W. Burkepile Jr.	1964 - 1970
	1972 - 1975
Gilbert E. Castree	1978 -
Orlando Diefenderfer	1972 - 1974
Harry S. Diehl	1965 - 1971
Daniel D. Dressler	1940 - 1946
Dr. Tamar D. Earnest	1987 - 1988
Robert D. Edwards	1976 -
Charles H. Esser	1954 - 1959
Jacob W. Esser	1961 -
Dr. Harold E. Everett	1975 - 1988
Rev. Charles E. Fair	1970 - 1975
	1978 - 1980
Tilghman G. Fenstermaker	1956 - 1981
Rev. Dr. Lester E. Fetter	1954 - 1961
Henry H. Fetterman	1945 - 1962
Rev. Dr. William A. Fluck	1957 - 1963
James J. Frankenfield	1980 - 1985
Russell E. Fulford	1957 - 1977
Harold G. Fulmer III	1983 - 1983
Rev. Gilbert B. Furst	1987 -
Rev. Waldemar L. Gallenkamp	1952 - 1955
David A. Gearhart	1981 -
Rev. Dr. George Gebert	1917 - 1940
Rev. Dr. G. Franklin Gehr	1936 - 1960
Rev. Dr. George A. Greiss	1932 - 1950
William O. Gross	1949 - 1967

John G. Guthrie	1976 - 1983
George M. Haddad	1976 - 1977
Rev. Dr. Maynard C. Hallock	1968 - 1973
Edna S. Hart	1930 - 1949
Rev. Ralph R. Hartzell	1948 - 1958
Rev. Warren C. Heinly	1945 - 1949
Judge James F. Henninger	1930 - 1961
Donald D. Hoffman	1986 -
Raymond E. Holland	1987 -
Thomas B. Hollenbach	1936 - 1956
John Raker Hudders	1979 -
Rev. Ira W. Klick	1909 - 1918
Rev. Dr. Richard Klick	1941 - 1961
Dr. Charles L. Knecht	1984 -
Robert W. Knipe	1981 -
Rev. Victor A. Kroninger Jr.	1978 - 1980
Ernest W. Kuhnsman	1974 - 1977
Robert W. Kurtz	1909 - 1924
	1940 - 1944
Rev. Dr. James Lambert	1924 - 1950
Rev. Ellerslie A. Lebo	1944 - 1953
Rev. Elmer E. Leisy	1949 - 1958
Paul E. Lentz	1971 - 1980
Peter W. Likins, Ph.D.	1987 -
Walter L. Lueke	1979 - 1985
A. J. Meyers	1930 - 1949
Rev. Curtis Miller	1930 - 1935
Rev. Harry P. Miller	1918 - 1927
Midge Mosser	1981 -
Robert K. Mosser	1941 - 1964
William F. Mosser Sr.	1954 - 1977
C. D. Moyer	1950 - 1953
Dr. Arlington Naugle	1962 - 1964
Julian W. Newhart	1970 -
Rev. S. E. Ochsenford	1922 - 1930
Dr. Walter J. Okunski	1988 -
Rev. Dr. Henry J. P. Pflum	1957 - 1963
Leonard P. Pool	1969 - 1974
Charles E. Radcliffe	1962 - 1967
Rev. Dr. Conrad W. Raker	1941 - 1980
D. Estella Raker	1909 - 1915
Rev. Dr. John H. Raker	1909 - 1941

William D. Reimert	1964 - 1969
Rev. Charles Ruloff	1961 - 1965
Pauline M. MacDonald Ruloff	1979 -
Rev. Dale Sandstrom	1980 -
Rev. Luther N. Schaeffer	1950 - 1979
Judge Henry V. Scheirer	1962 - 1980
Rev. Dr. Theodore C. Schlack	1981 - 1985
Rev. Ernest G. Schmidt	1968 - 1973
Leonard Sefing Jr.	1909 - 1909
Kristi L. Shafer	1983 -
Elmer K. Shaffer	1962 - 1968
Rev. Dr. Francis A. Shearer	1941 - 1947
Rev. Harvey C. Snyder	1950 - 1956
Frank E. Speer	1965 - 1970
Augustus Stang Jr.	1974 - 1979
Rev. Samuel F. Stauffer	1970 - 1973
John H. Stiles	1941 - 1945
Dr. Clifford H. Trexler	1971 - 1973
Peter S. Trumbower	1931 - 1944
Rev. Dr. William Wackernagel	1909 - 1926
Rev. M. Luther Wahrmann	1959 - 1962
Rev. Dr. Conrad Wilker	1930 - 1944
Charles S. Wingert	1965 - 1967
Rev. Richard C. Wolf	1975 -
Rev. Hugh E. Yost	1964 - 1978
Elsie C. Ziegler	1962 - 1964

DATES

Jan. 1, 1863	John H. Raker born.
June 5, 1879	D. Estella Weiser born.
June 5, 1899	John H. Raker - D. Estella Weiser wed.
Dec. 4, 1907	Viola Raker dies.
Feb. 21, 1908	Home founded, Viola Hunt admitted.
Feb. 25, 1908	Kline Homestead purchased.
Aug. 26, 1909	Ladies Auxiliary founded.
Nov. 9, 1909	Board incorporated by court.
May 13, 1910	Constitution adopted.
Aug. 4, 1910	Infants cottage purchased.
Apr. 21, 1911	Old folks cottage bought.
Oct. 27, 1912	Conrad W. Raker born.
Mar. 21, 1915	Farms purchased in Salisbury Township.
July 18, 1918	601 St. John Street purchased.
Aug. 23, 1923	New boys' dorm dedicated.
June 24, 1933	Dale Sandstrom born.
June 1, 1937	Conrad Raker named assistant.
Sept. 25, 1938	Dispensary dedicated.
May 8, 1941	John H. Raker dies.
Sept. 10, 1941	Conrad Raker named superintendent.
1944	Home's value exceeds $1 million.
Aug. 22, 1948	Conrad Raker - Hannah (Ely) Jacks wed.
Aug. 11, 1962	D. Estella (Weiser) Raker dies.
June 28, 1964	Rehabilitation Center groundbreaking.
June 6, 1965	Rehabilitation Center dedication.
1968	Year's operating expenses top $1 million.
Oct. 8, 1968	Herman E. C. Warhmann dies at 98.
Sept. 6, 1978	Dale Sandstrom named assistant.
Mar. 26, 1980	Conrad Raker resigns as administrator. Dale Sandstrom becomes administrator.

Apr. 3, 1980	Hannah (Ely) Raker dies.
Aug. 17, 1980	Raker Center dedicated.
July 31, 1983	Rehabilitation Hospital dedicated.
May 21, 1986	Conrad Raker - Grace (Jordan) Moritz wed.
Apr. 19, 1988	Robert and Marian Edwards Center dedicated.
July 10, 1988	Berger, Brubaker and Youngdahl wings dedicated.

GOOD SHEPHERD
REHABILITATION HOSPITAL SERVICES

Proclaiming itself as "one of America's most comprehensive rehabilitation facilities," the hospital offered the following services in Good Shepherd's 80th anniversary year:

Academic education
Activities of daily living training
Amputee clinic
Architectural home evaluation
Arthritis pool program
Audiology
Back school
Burn rehabilitation
Cardiopulmonary rehabilitation program
Case management
Children's diagnostic center
Chronic pain management
Community re-entry
Comprehensive arthritis rehabilitation program
Consulting services (medical and management)
Comprehensive outpatient rehabilitation facilities
Counseling
Day care center for children
Diagnostic laboratory
Driver evaluation and training
Electrodiagnostic evaluation
Ergonomic engineering

Ergonomic jobsite analysis
Expert witness
Hand rehabilitation
Head injury program
Independent living training
Industrial consultation services
Industrial fitness program
Industrial medicine
Industrial services
Injured worker management
Injury prevention program.
Inpatient rehabilitation hospital
Internships
Low back program
Long term care
Multiple sclerosis clinic
Muscular Dystrophy Association clinic
Neuropsychological assessment
Occupational therapy
Orthopedic services
Orthotic clinic and services
Outpatient therapy centers
Pain management program

Pastoral services
Pediatric rehabilitation
Physiatric evaluations
Physical capacities
    evaluations
Physical work capacities
    evaluations
Physical therapy
Pre-employment
    evaluations
Prosthetic/orthotic
    fabrication
Psychological evaluation
    and treatment
Punchclock rehabilitation
Rehabilitation client and
    family support groups
Rehabilitation
    engineering
Rehabilitation medicine
    and nursing

Scoliosis rehabilitation
Sexuality education
Social work services
Speech and
    communication therapy
Spinal cord injury
    program
Stroke re-entry group
Therapeutic pool
Therapeutic recreation
Urodynamics studies
Vocational rehabilitation
Wheelchair prescription
    and repair
Wholistic health care
Work capacities
    assessment
Workers' compensation
Work hardening
X-ray

311

312

316